Individualized Diabetes Management

A Guide for Primary Care

D1471798

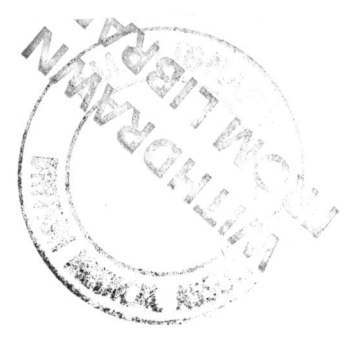

Individualized Diabetes Management

A Guide for Primary Care

Anthony H. Barnett
Jenny Grice

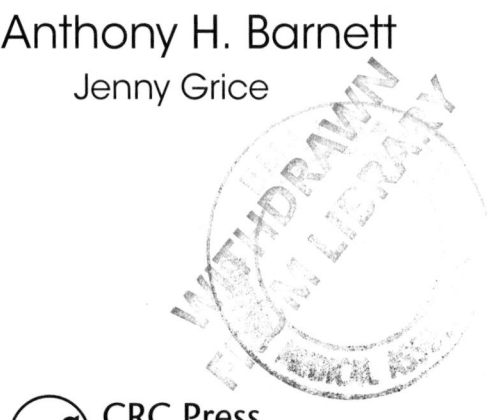

CRC Press
Taylor & Francis Group
Boca Raton London New York

CRC Press is an imprint of the
Taylor & Francis Group, an **informa** business

CRC Press
Taylor & Francis Group
6000 Broken Sound Parkway NW, Suite 300
Boca Raton, FL 33487-2742

© 2016 by Taylor & Francis Group, LLC
CRC Press is an imprint of Taylor & Francis Group, an Informa business

No claim to original U.S. Government works

Printed on acid-free paper
Version Date: 20160719
Printed at CPI on sustainably sourced paper

International Standard Book Number-13: 978-1-4987-6209-0 (Paperback)

Library of Congress Cataloging-in-Publication Data

Names: Barnett, A. H. (Anthony H.), 1951- author. | Grice, Jenny, author.
Title: Individualized diabetes management : a guide for primary care /
Anthony H. Barnett and Jenny Grice.
Description: Boca Raton : CRC Press, [2017] | Includes bibliographical
references.
Identifiers: LCCN 2016032387 | ISBN 9781498762090 (pbk. : alk. paper)
Subjects: | MESH: Diabetes Mellitus, Type 2-- epidemiology | Diabetes
Mellitus, Type 2--therapy | Precision Medicine | Primary Health Care |
Great Britain
Classification: LCC RC660.4 | NLM WK 810 | DDC 616.4/62-- dc23
LC record available at https://lccn.loc.gov/2016032387

Visit the Taylor & Francis Web site at
http://www.taylorandfrancis.com

and the CRC Press Web site at
http://www.crcpress.com

Contents

Biography

Professor Anthony H. Barnett is recognised as an international expert in this area and has written many papers and lectured extensively nationally and abroad. He has acted as an expert advisor to National Institute for Health and Care Excellence (NICE) on new drugs and has worked with the European Medicines Agency and other related bodies. Indeed, he represented the European Association for the Study of Diabetes (EASD) at the European Medicines Agency on diabetes-related drugs between 2006 and 2011. He is presently listed in the top five researchers in Type 2 Diabetes worldwide.

Jenny Grice is an accomplished medical writer and has supported Professor Barnett on many of his projects including co-authoring a bespoke book on new mechanisms in glucose control, published in 2011.

Introduction

Type 2 diabetes is at crisis levels and shows no signs of abating with no country and no section of society immune to the disease. In the United Kingdom, 2016 began with the news that the number of people with diabetes had exceeded four million for the first time (QOF et al., 2015). The need to tackle this serious health condition has therefore never been so urgent.

Although we have the evidence and the tools to prevent and manage type 2 diabetes, these are not routinely employed, and tragically we continue to see too many people with diabetes suffering serious complications, and even premature death. The challenge is to reduce the human and financial costs through early diagnosis and effective management and to prevent new cases of diabetes from developing.

The World Innovation Summit for Health 2015 Diabetes Forum identified three policy goals to both reduce the incidence of diabetes and better manage established disease and its complications (Colagiuri et al., 2015):

1. Improve disease management for people with diabetes to reduce complication rates.
2. Establish effective surveillance to identify and support those at risk of type 2 diabetes.
3. Introduce a range of interventions that help to create an environment focussed on prevention.

IMPROVE DISEASE MANAGEMENT

In the past two decades, a greater understanding of diabetes has facilitated the development of new drug classes that target specific metabolic pathways such as the thiazolidinediones, dipeptidyl peptidase-4 inhibitors, glucagon-like peptide-1 receptor agonists and sodium–glucose cotransporter type 2 inhibitors, as well as a range of new insulins (Tahrani et al., 2016). Many of these are now available as combination treatments allowing us to combine drugs with different mechanisms of action into simpler treatment regimens. We are no longer limited in what we can offer to patients, and it is therefore much easier to develop personalised management regimens that match treatments to the individual needs of patients and their stage of disease. The clinical efficacy of a treatment remains integral, but what is more important to the individual is how it fits in with his or her daily life, and here ease of use, tolerability and safety are of great importance. Tailored treatment plans combined with education improve disease management and help prevent complications.

Unless personalised management plans suited to the needs of the individual and well supported by health care professionals are applied consistently, the rising number of people with diabetes will have less chance of living long and healthy lives, and health authorities will become crippled by the avoidable but escalating costs of treating poorly managed diabetes and its many sequelae. It should be remembered that the cost of best practice management, including appropriate drug therapy in diabetes, is a small proportion of the total cost (most of which is accounted for by the often preventable long-term complications). It is entirely paradoxical, therefore, to withhold best practice management from patients earlier in the disease ostensibly to reduce costs if in the long term this leads to an increased risk of complications, which account for the vast majority of the costs of type 2 diabetes. The latter relate to significantly increased risk of blindness, kidney failure, lower limb amputation, myocardial infarction and stroke. All too often we (and particularly health authorities) consider the headline 'cost' of a management regime (particularly as it relates to drug therapy) rather than its true value.

IDENTIFY THOSE AT RISK

Although there is as yet no cure, type 2 diabetes is largely preventable – both its onset and its complications. The most important modifiable risk factors for type 2 diabetes are overweight and obesity, which have now reached massive proportions in both the developed countries and the developing world (Aylott et al., 2008). Indeed, there has been a fourfold increase in the prevalence of obesity in UK adults over the past 30 years with similar worrying statistics in children and young people (Aylott et al., 2008). Levels of physical activity have plummeted in a generation, and the 'fast food' culture has taken over.

Primary care is ideally placed to become more directly involved in diabetes prevention, although this must be supported by appropriate public health initiatives and resources. We can identify people at risk of developing type 2 diabetes by looking at their family history, their ethnicity, their weight, how active they are and what their diet is like, and offer education and support to those at risk. We can also identify those people with type 2 diabetes who are not managing well and focus more resources on these individuals. This will potentially help enormously in the overall cost of care, by reducing hospitalisations and complications.

CREATE A PREVENTION-FOCUSED ENVIRONMENT

This last point is less in the hands of primary care and more in those of policy makers. To create an environment that encourages healthy living and prevents diabetes, policymakers need to address risk factors rather than focus solely on the disease. This requires a wide variety of interventions to change population behaviour.

In addition, with the record number of people living with diabetes, there is no time to waste in improving diabetes care and education. Every delay in diagnosis and treatment can lead to more complications and more suffering for patients as well as a huge financial cost to the National Health Service. The increasing requirement in the United Kingdom to move much of diabetes practice into the community means that primary care must take on much of this role. We know what needs to be done, the question is how to do it? In this bespoke book, the authors focus on how to personalise care and how advances in treatment are making this easier to achieve. Although there are many areas involved in individualised prescribing and management, the book focuses on those that are within the control of the person with diabetes and his or her healthcare provider. These include helping people with diabetes gain the skills to manage their own health, agreeing with them a care plan that is based on their personal needs, and making sure that their care is better coordinated. Tackling diabetes is one of the major health challenges of our time. By ensuring that action is taken now to offer the best possible care for diabetes, this will be repaid, in human, social and economic terms, but will require substantial commitment from all those involved.

REFERENCES

Aylott J, Brown I, Copeland R, Johnson D. Tackling obesities: The foresight report and implications for local government. Sheffield Hallam University; 2008. Available from: http://www.idea.gov.uk/idk/aio/8268011. Last accessed May 2011.

Colagiuri S, Kent J, Kainu T, Sutherland S, Vui S; World Innovation Summit for Health. Rising to the Challenge Preventing and Managing Type 2 Diabetes Report of the WISH Diabetes Forum 2015; 2015. Available from: https://www.imperial.ac.uk/media/imperial-college/institute-of-global-health-innovation/public/Diabetes.pdf. Last accessed March 2016.

Quality and Outcomes Framework, Health and Social Care Information Centre, Information Services Division Scotland. *Statistics for Wales*. Department of Health, Social Services and Public Safety; 2014–2015.

Tahrani AA, Barnett AH, Bailey CJ. Pharmacology and therapeutic implications of current drugs for type 2 diabetes mellitus. *Nat Rev Endocrinol* 2016;12:566–592.

1

Type 2 diabetes: epidemiology, complications and costs

EPIDEMIOLOGY

Changes in lifestyle over the past century have resulted in a dramatic increase in the incidence of type 2 diabetes worldwide. Once a disease of Western affluent societies, it has now spread to every country in the world and is increasingly common among the poor. Once almost unheard of in children, rising rates of childhood obesity have rendered it more common in the paediatric population, especially in certain ethnic groups. Recent estimates from the Global Burden of Disease Study indicate that diabetes rates around the world rose 45% between 1990 and 2013, primarily in type 2 diabetes (Global Burden of Disease Study 2013 Collaborators, 2015). According to the International Diabetes Federation, diabetes affected at least 387 million people worldwide in 2014, and that number is expected to rise to 592 million by 2035, with 77% of all diabetes cases occurring in low- to middle-income countries (IDF, 2015).

China and India now account for 60% of the world's diabetes population. In 1980, less than 1% of Chinese adults had diabetes, but this increased to almost 12% (113.9 million adults) by 2010 (Diabetes in China, 2014). The epidemic is the result of rapid economic development, urbanization and lifestyles that are increasingly sedentary, and poor diets high in saturated fat and calories derived from refined carbohydrates and sugar. Asian people are also particularly susceptible to type 2 diabetes compared with white people and tend to develop the disease at a much lower body mass index (BMI). The average BMI of Chinese people with diabetes is 25 kg/m^2, compared with 30 kg/m^2 in non-Asians.

Recent prevalence figures for the United Kingdom have been obtained using data from the Quality and Outcomes Framework for those aged ≥17 years and the National Paediatric Diabetes Audit for England and Wales and the Scottish Diabetes Survey for younger individuals. The data show that at the end of March 2014, there were approximately three million people with a recorded diagnosis of type 2 diabetes, which equates to a prevalence of 4.5% (Table 1.1) (Holman et al., 2015). Throughout the United Kingdom, 1 in 22 people have diagnosed type 2 diabetes. However, these figures do not take into account the numbers of people with undiagnosed type 2 diabetes, currently estimated at around 850,000 (Public Health England, 2014a).

Overweight and obesity are driving the global diabetes epidemic. They affect the majority of adults in most developed countries and are increasing rapidly in developing countries. In the United Kingdom, around 90% of people with type 2 diabetes are overweight or obese (Public Health England, 2014b). The rising prevalence of obesity in the United Kingdom and around the world will continue to lead to a rise in the prevalence of type 2 diabetes. It is estimated that at least half of all cases of type 2 diabetes could be prevented if weight gain in adults could be avoided (Knowler et al., 2002). As a consequence, an epidemic of diabetes-related complications and premature mortality will follow, with people from deprived areas and some minority ethnic groups at particularly high risk.

Table 1.1 Current prevalence of diagnosed diabetes in the United Kingdom

	Type of diabetes					
	Type 1		Type 2		Other	
	Number of people	Prevalence (%)	Number of people	Prevalence (%)	Number of people	Prevalence (%)
England	235,163	0.4	2,567,439	4.6	33,679	0.06
Wales	13,926	0.4	162,738	5.1	1,957	0.06
Scotland	28,319	0.5	231,871	4.3	2,447	0.05
Great Britain	277,408	0.4	2,962,049	4.6	38,082	0.06
Northern Ireland[a]	6,997	0.4	74,712	3.9	961	0.05
The United Kingdom	284,405	0.4	3,036,761	4.5	39,043	0.06

Source: Adapted from Holman, N. et al., Diabet Med, 32, 1119–1120, 2015.

[a] Estimated based on the breakdown of the type of diagnosed diabetes in Great Britain.

DIABETES COMPLICATIONS

Diabetes is a chronic disease that causes substantial premature morbidity and death. Over time, damage caused by high blood glucose levels is a major contributing factor to long-term complications, which can be classified broadly as microvascular (including retinopathy, nephropathy and neuropathy) (Figure 1.1) or macrovascular disease (including ischaemic heart disease, myocardial infarction, heart failure and stroke). Without careful, continued management of the condition, a person with diabetes faces a reduced life expectancy of between 6 and 20 years (The Emerging Risk Factors Collaboration, 2011). According to a report conducted by the Health & Social Care Information Centre in 2013, there were around 24,000 premature deaths in England and Wales due to diabetes (both type 1 and type 2) compared to the general population. Those with type 1 diabetes were 131% more likely to die in 2013 than their peers without the condition, and those with type 2 diabetes were 32% more likely to die (National Diabetes Audit: Complications and mortality, 2015). These additional deaths are largely preventable and develop after years of exposure to high glucose, high blood pressure and high cholesterol, which are all signs of poorly managed diabetes. The report

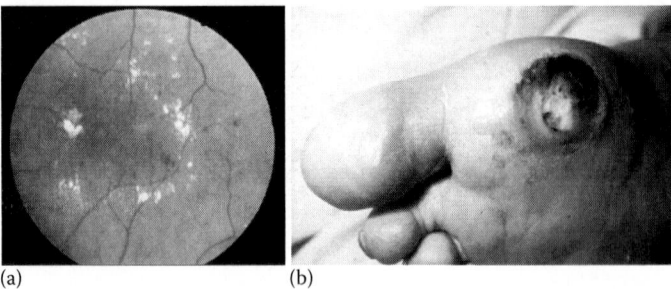

(a)   (b)

Figure 1.1 Examples of type 2 diabetes associated microvascular complications, including retinopathy and neuropathic ulcer. (a) Hard exudates are visible gathering around the macular region of the retina suggestive of sight threatening maculopathy. Retinal microaneurysms can also be seen. (b) Neuropathic ulcer over the metatarsal head of the big toe.

assessed the likelihood of a person with diabetes being admitted to hospital for each of a range of diabetes complications, including angina, myocardial infarction, heart failure, stroke, major amputation, minor amputation and renal replacement therapy (dialysis or transplantation). Compared to a person without diabetes, people with diabetes were significantly more likely to be admitted to hospital with one of the complications (Figure 1.2) (National Diabetes Audit: Complications and mortality, 2015).

The increasing prevalence of type 2 diabetes in younger adults will also have an impact on the incidence of diabetes complications. In the United Kingdom, the proportion of newly diagnosed people with type 2 diabetes below the age of 40 years has increased significantly from 5.9% in 1991 to 12.4% in 2010 (Holden et al., 2013). A diagnosis of type 2 diabetes at a young age will lead to the development of complications at an earlier stage of life, and indeed there is evidence that young-onset diabetes is a more aggressive disease

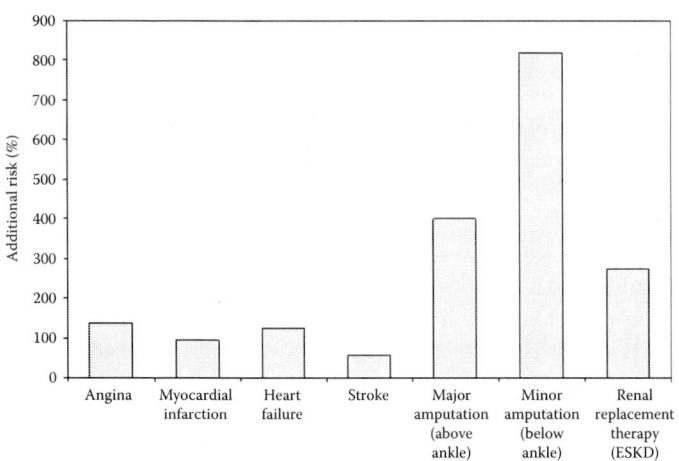

Figure 1.2 Additional risk of a person with diabetes being admitted to hospital for each of a range of diabetes complications compared to somebody without diabetes over a 1-year follow-up period using the 2011–2012 National Diabetes Audit. (Adapted from National Diabetes Audit—2012–2013. Report 2: Complications and mortality. Available from: http://www.hscic.gov.uk/catalogue/PUB16496/nati-diab-audi-12-13-rep2.pdf, 2015.)

than that occurring in older people (Rhodes et al., 2012). Preventing vascular complications from occurring would therefore have a huge impact on the number of hospital admissions across the National Health Service (NHS). In the United Kingdom, the National Institute for Health and Care Excellence (NICE) already recommends screening for diabetes in high-risk individuals aged 25–39 years particularly from ethnic minority groups and those with conditions that increase the risk of type 2 diabetes (NICE, 2012).

There is also now a substantial body of epidemiological evidence to suggest that intrauterine exposure to hyperglycaemia is associated with increased lifelong risks of the exposed offspring for obesity, metabolic, cardiovascular and malignant diseases. During early development, the foetus is particularly vulnerable to environmental factors, and that to benefit the next generation avoiding adverse nutrition during the pre-conception and intrauterine period may be much more important for the prevention of adult disease than preventive measures in infants and adults (Lehnen et al., 2013).

COSTS

With its increasing prevalence and high cost of treatment, diabetes places an enormous demand on economic resources. In 1993, the cost of diabetes treatment in China was 2.2 billion (bn) Renminbi (RMB), but the projected cost for 2030 is 360 bn RMB. In the United States, it is estimated that approximately 20% of the nation's healthcare budget goes towards treating people with diabetes (ADA, 2013). In Europe, preventing and treating diabetes and its complications is estimated to cost about 90 bn euros (£73 bn) annually. In the United Kingdom, treating people with diabetes and its complications cost the NHS £8.8 bn in 2010–2011, equivalent to around 10% of the NHS budget. By 2035, it is predicted that costs will have increased to £16.8 bn, 17% of the NHS entire budget.

The cost impact of diabetes affects society, health systems, individuals and employers, and reflects both direct costs of the disease such as doctor and hospital visits, medication, laboratory costs for tests and equipment costs, and indirect costs such as income losses due to reduced employment chances, early retirement and lost work hours due to illness. Many people with type 2 diabetes experience multiple complications, compounding the complexity of treatment and thus costs. The characteristics of the economic burden vary from country to country depending on the health-care system in place. In high-income countries, the burden often affects government or public health insurance budgets, whereas in low- and middle-income countries, where about two-thirds of all individuals with diabetes live, a large part of the burden falls on the person with diabetes and their family due to limited or no health insurance coverage (Seuring et al., 2015).

In 2014/2015, the net ingredient cost for managing diabetes in the United Kingdom was £868.6 million, according to the NHS prescription data group the Health and Social Care Information Centre. This represents 10% of the total primary care prescribing spend, that is, 10 pence in the pound of the primary care prescribing bill in England is being spent on managing diabetes. However, around four-fifths of NHS diabetes spending goes on treating complications that in many cases could have been prevented. In a recent analysis from the UK Prospective Diabetes Study (UKPDS), the costs of all consultations, visits, admissions and procedures associated with diabetes-related complications during the UKPDS post-trial monitoring period (1997–2007) were estimated using hospital records for 2791 patients and resource use questionnaires administered to 3589 patients (Alva et al., 2015). Using the example of a 60-year-old man, the estimated inpatient costs (during the event year) were as follows: £9767 for non-fatal ischaemic heart disease; £3766 for fatal ischaemic heart disease; £6379 for non-fatal myocardial infarction; £1521 for fatal myocardial infarction; £3191 for heart failure; £6805 for non-fatal stroke; £3954 for fatal stroke; £9546 for amputation; and £1355 for blindness in one eye. Given the fact that most of these complications are preventable, the costs are wasteful not only in terms of the quality of human life, but also for NHS budgets. If nothing is done to halt this epidemic, the double burden of an ageing population and rising rates of young-onset type 2 diabetes will have an enormous toll on productivity and healthcare systems. Long-term cost savings can only be achieved if urgent measures are put in place to ensure early investment into prevention and better disease management.

REFERENCES

Diabetes in China: mapping the road ahead. Lancet *Diabetes Endocrinol* 2014;2:923.

Alva ML, Gray A, Mihaylova B, Leal J, Holman RR. The impact of diabetes-related complications on healthcare costs: New results from the UKPDS (UKPDS 84). *Diabetic Med* 2015;32:459–466.

American Diabetes Association. Economic costs of diabetes in the U.S. in 2012. *Diabetes Care* 2013;36:1033–1046.

The Emerging Risk Factors Collaboration. Diabetes mellitus, fasting glucose, and risk of cause-specific death. *N Engl J Med* 2011;364:829–841.

Global Burden of Disease Study 2013 Collaborators. Global, regional, and national incidence, prevalence, and years lived with disability for 301 acute and chronic diseases and injuries in 188 countries, 1990–2013: A systematic analysis for the Global Burden of Disease Study 2013. *Lancet* 2015;386:743–800.

Holden SH, Barnett AH, Peters JR, Jenkins-Jones S, Poole CD, Morgan CL, Currie CJ. The incidence of type 2 diabetes in the United Kingdom from 1991 to 2010. *Diabetes Obes Metab* 2013;15:8448–8452.

Holman N, Young B, Gadsby R. Current prevalence of Type 1 and Type 2 diabetes in adults and children in the UK. *Diabet Med* 2015;32:1119–1120.

International Diabetes Federation. *IDF Diabetes Atlas. Epidemiology and Mobidity*; 2015. Available from http://www.idf.org/. Last accessed 1 March 2016.

Knowler WC, Barrett-Connor E, Fowler SE, Hamman RF, Lachin JM, Walker EA, Nathan DM; Diabetes Prevention Program Research Group. Reduction in the incidence of type 2 diabetes with lifestyle intervention or metformin. *N Engl J Med* 2002 Feb 7;346(6):393–403.

Lehnen H, Zechner U, Haaf T. Epigenetics of gestational diabetes mellitus and offspring health: The time for action is in early stages of life. *Mol Hum Reprod* 2013;19:415–422.

National Diabetes Audit—2012–2013. Report 2: Complications and Mortality. Available from: http://www.hscic.gov.uk/catalogue/PUB16496/nati-diab-audi-12-13-rep2.pdf. Last accessed November 2015.

NICE. *Preventing type 2 diabetes: Risk identification and interventions for individuals at high risk.* London: National Institute for Health and Care Excellence; 2012.

Public Health England. Diabetes prevalence model 2014a. Available from: http://www.yhpho.org.uk/resource/view.aspx?RID=81090. Last accessed 28 September 2016.

Public Health England. Adult obesity and type 2 diabetes 2014b. Available from: https://www.gov.uk/government/uploads/system/uploads/attachment_data/file/338934/Adult_obesity_and_type_2_diabetes.pdf. Last accessed 28 September 2016.

Rhodes ET, Prosser LA, Hoerger TJ, et al. Estimated morbidity and mortality in adolescents and young adults diagnosed with type 2 diabetes mellitus. *Diabet Med* 2012;29:453–463.

Seuring T, Archangelidi O, Suhrcke M. The economic costs of type 2 diabetes: A global systematic review. *Pharmacoeconomics* 2015;33:811–831.

2

Challenges to glycaemic control

Achieving and maintaining adequate glycaemic control remains a challenge in many people with type 2 diabetes. The most recent National Institute for Health and Care Excellence (NICE) guidelines recommend second-line intervention if haemoglobin A1c (HbA1c) rises to 7.5% (58 mmol/mol) or higher with a combination of reinforced lifestyle advice and intensified drug treatment. HbA1c treatment targets are personalised, but in general should be 6.5% (48 mmol/mol) for diet ± metformin and 7% (53 mmol/mol) after intensification beyond this (National Institute for Health and Care Excellence, 2015). Statistics from the UK National Diabetes Audit for 2014/2015 indicate that around one-third of individuals with a diagnosis of type 2 diabetes in England and Wales have an HbA1c higher than 7.5% (58 mmol/mol) (National Diabetes Audit, 2014/2015) (Table 2.1), a figure that has hardly changed in the past 5 years. The proportion of people with a serum cholesterol level higher than NICE recommendations has remained stable, whereas blood pressure target achievement rates have improved steadily (Table 2.1).

The maintenance of simultaneous control of hypertension, dyslipidaemia and hyperglycaemia is the cornerstone of diabetes care, but this was achieved in only 41% of individuals (Table 2.1) (achievements would have been even less if 'best practice' targets had been audited, that is, HbA1c <7% [53 mmol/mol], blood

Table 2.1 Percentage of people with diabetes in England and Wales achieving their treatment targets by diabetes type and audit year

	Type 1					Type 2 and other				
	2010–2011	2011–2012	2012–2013	2013–2014	2014–2015	2010–2011	2011–2012	2012–2013	2013–2014	2014–2015
HbA1c ≤58 mmol/mol	28.1	27.0	27.2	29.4	29.9	66.5	65.8	64.9	66.8	66.1
Blood pressure ≤140/80 mmHg	68.8	72.2	73.4	76.4	76.4	61.4	66.6	68.6	73.6	74.2
Cholesterol <5 mmol/L	72.0	71.1	70.2	71.5	71.5	78.0	77.4	76.7	77.8	77.5
Meeting all three treatment targets	16.5	16.5	16.1	18.6	18.9	35.1	37.4	37.3	41.4	41.0

Source: Adapted from National Diabetes Audit—2013–2014 and 2014–2015: Report 1, Care processes and treatment targets. Available from: http://www.hscic.gov.uk/catalogue/PUB19900/nati-diab-rep1-audi-2013-15.pdf.

pressure <130/80 mmHg and total and low-density lipoprotein (LDL) cholesterol <4 and 2 mmol/L, respectively). Compared with its European counterparts, the United Kingdom appears better at managing lipids and blood pressure than hyperglycaemia. In a cross-sectional study that examined the medical records of people with type 2 diabetes across eight European countries over the period March 2009–December 2010, the United Kingdom was second lowest in terms of HbA1c target attainment (defined as an HbA1c <7% [53 mmol/mol]) (Table 2.2) (Stone et al., 2013).

According to the National Diabetes Audit, people aged 65 and over were more likely to achieve simultaneous control of hypertension, dyslipidaemia and hyperglycaemia (just under 50% achieved control) compared with individuals aged 40–64 years old where only a third achieved control (Figure 2.1) (National Diabetes Audit, 2014/2015).

Managing type 2 diabetes appropriately is critical to control its progression and to prevent acute and long-term complications, which are not only detrimental to quality of life and long-term prognosis, but also account for a disproportionate share of the total cost of managing the condition (Liebl et al., 2015). Three main factors continue to challenge glycaemic control: the progressive nature of the disease, poor adherence to management plans and clinical inertia ('the deadly triad') (Figure 2.2).

TYPE 2 DIABETES IS A PROGRESSIVE DISEASE

Two major pathophysiological abnormalities underlie most cases of type 2 diabetes: insulin resistance (impaired insulin sensitivity) and β-cell dysfunction. As cells and organs become gradually less sensitive to insulin, the body tries to compensate by producing more insulin, and also by increasing the number of insulin-secreting β-cells. When insulin resistance is accompanied by β-cell dysfunction, failure to control blood glucose levels results. Both abnormalities are essential components of type 2 diabetes pathogenesis, but it is the progressive loss of β-cell function that is central to the progression of the disease.

The management of type 2 diabetes can be considered a 'moving target,' in that the underlying pathophysiology is constantly

Table 2.2 Achievement of type 2 diabetes treatment targets across eight European countries

Target	Percentage (95% confidence intervals) meeting target							
	Belgium	France	Germany	Ireland	Italy	The Netherlands	Sweden	The United Kingdom
HbA1c <7%	59.7	65.3	48.6	53.4	35.7	70.5	56.5	39.1
(53 mmol/mol)	(56.7–62.8)	(62.4–68.2)	(45.4–51.9)	(50.2–56.7)	(32.7–38.7)	(67.7–73.3)	(52.3–60.6)	(36.1–42.1)
BP (combined)	17.6	14.9	7.4	24.9	20.8	20.3	27.1	25.0
<130/80 mmHg	(15.3–20.0)	(12.7–17.1)	(5.7–9.1)	(22.1–27.8)	(18.2–23.3)	(17.9–22.8)	(23.3–30.8)	(22.3–27.7)
Total cholesterol	23.1	25.7	11.7	52.6	19.7	34.5	22.8	45.5
<4 mmol/L	(20.5–25.7)	(23.0–28.5)	(9.5–13.9)	(49.3–55.9)	(17.2–22.2)	(31.6–37.4)	(19.1–26.5)	(42.3–48.6)
LDL cholesterol	49.7	52.4	30.7	76.9	40.4	58.9	47.3	74.5
<2.6 mmol/L	(46.6–52.8)	(49.2–55.6)	(27.1–34.3)	(74.0–79.8)	(36.8–43.9)	(55.8–62.0)	(42.0–52.5)	(71.4–77.6)

Source: Adapted from Stone, M.A. et al., Diabetes Care, 36, 2628–2638, 2013.

Note: Data extracted retrospectively from medical records of people with type 2 diabetes between March 2009 and December 2010.

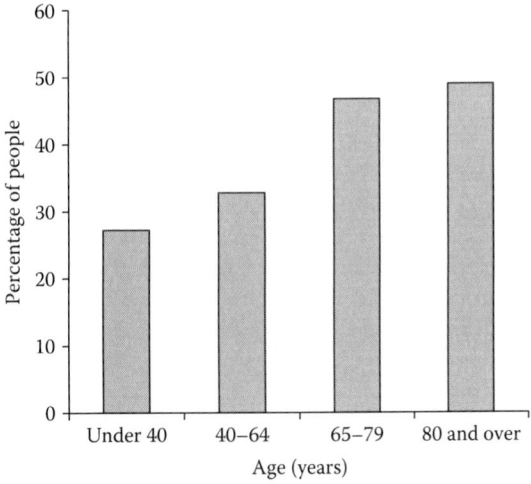

Figure 2.1 Percentage of people with type 2 diabetes in England and Wales achieving all three treatment targets (HbA1c $\leq$7.5% [58 mmol/mol], blood pressure $\leq$140/80 mmHg and cholesterol <5 mmol/L) by age group, 2014–2015. (Adapted from National Diabetes Audit—2013–2014 and 2014–2015: Report 1, Care processes and treatment targets. Available from: http://www.hscic.gov.uk/catalogue/PUB19900/nati-diab-rep1-audi-2013-15.pdf.)

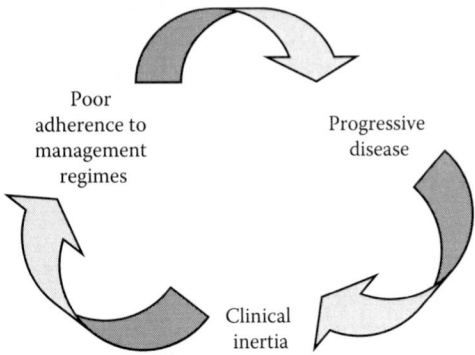

Figure 2.2 Challenges to good glycaemic control (all three are intimately interlinked).

changing and progressing. It is therefore unlikely to respond adequately to any single therapy in the long term, resulting in complex prescribing patterns as the disease progresses with regular adjustments required over time. Furthermore, individuals with type 2 diabetes vary in their levels of insulin resistance and β-cell dysfunction. This has important implications for disease management. For example, the more insulin resistant a person with type 2 diabetes is, the harder it is to manage the disease with agents whose mechanisms of action are insulin dependent because more medication is required to provide enough insulin to achieve target blood glucose levels. The management of type 2 diabetes therefore requires treatment that is personalised to specific glucose (and other cardiovascular risk factors) problems and other health conditions.

The risk of insulin resistance increases with age, and some individuals are genetically more susceptible. Lifestyle also plays a role, with a higher risk in overweight individuals and those with a sedentary lifestyle. A key feature of any diabetes management programme is therefore diet and exercise. Dietary carbohydrate is the major determinant of post-prandial glucose levels, and low carbohydrate diets can be effective for improving glycaemic control and achieving weight loss in people with type 2 diabetes (Ajala et al., 2013). Exercise can dramatically reduce insulin resistance. In addition to making the body more sensitive to insulin and building muscle that can absorb blood glucose, physical activity opens up an alternative pathway for glucose to enter muscle cells without insulin acting as an intermediary. This reduces the cells' dependence on insulin for energy. Although the latter does not reduce insulin resistance itself, it can help people who are insulin resistant improve their blood glucose control.

Guidelines stress the importance of diet and exercise in the treatment of all stages of type 2 diabetes. These lifestyle measures are cheap and have no long-term side effects, but they demand a high degree of motivation, which will require ongoing support. Many people will require intensification of therapy to oral anti-diabetes agents and the early initiation of combination treatment if glycaemic control is not achieved.

ADHERENCE TO MANAGEMENT PLANS

Adherence to treatments for type 2 diabetes is complicated by the fact that individuals often need to take multiple medications for their diabetes and concurrent conditions, with different dosage frequencies and varying numbers of tablets at different times of the day. The overall management of type 2 diabetes should therefore address treatment adherence as well as appropriate medications (although the two are very much interlinked). Drug and lifestyle measures to control type 2 diabetes and associated conditions can only be effective through adherence to the overall prescribed regimen. When intensifying treatment regimens, it is therefore important to consider how this can be achieved without reducing adherence.

Reasons for non-adherence are multifactorial and factors may include age, lack of information, perception and duration of disease, complexity of dosing regimen, polypharmacy, psychological factors, tolerability (probably the single most important factor) and, in some countries, cost. Various measures to increase patient satisfaction and adherence in type 2 diabetes have been investigated. These include reducing the complexity of therapy by using fixed-dose combination pills and less frequent dosing regimens, using medications that are associated with fewer adverse events (hypoglycaemia or weight gain), educational initiatives with improved patient–healthcare provider communication and reminder systems. A more detailed discussion of the barriers to adherence and potential solutions is provided in Chapter 3.

CLINICAL INERTIA

Clinical inertia is defined as the failure to initiate or intensify therapy despite an inadequate treatment response and has multiple causes relating to providers, patients and the healthcare system (Figure 2.3). It contributes to inadequate disease care in diabetes as well as a number of other chronic diseases, including hypertension, dyslipidaemia, depression and coronary heart disease. One report states that the contribution of clinical inertia is as likely to cause adverse clinical outcomes as medical errors,

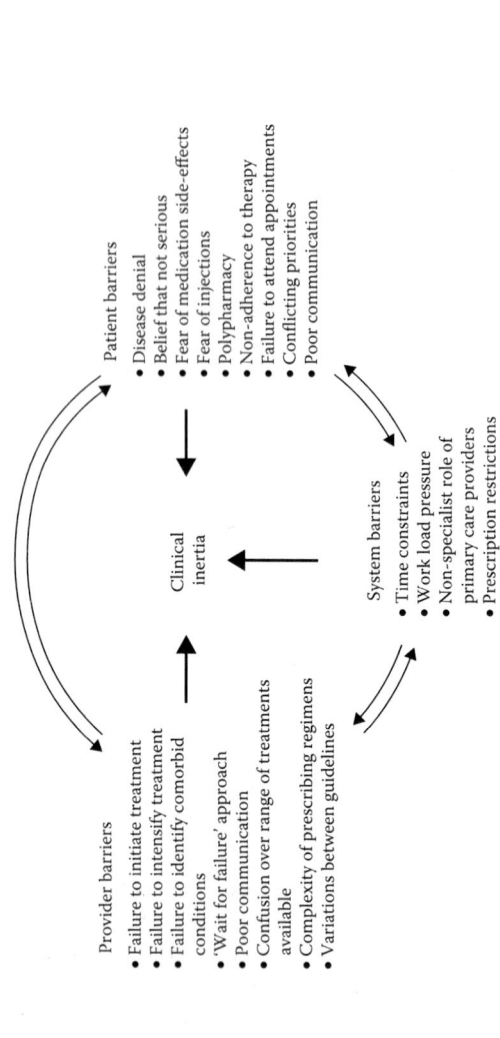

Figure 2.3 Conceptual model illustrating the contribution of provider, patient and system barriers to clinical inertia and how they interlink. (Adapted from O'Connor, P.J. et al., *Advances in Patient Safety: From Research to Implementation*, Agency for Healthcare Research and Quality (US), Rockville, Maryland, 2005.)

Patient barriers
- Disease denial
- Belief that not serious
- Fear of medication side-effects
- Fear of injections
- Polypharmacy
- Non-adherence to therapy
- Failure to attend appointments
- Conflicting priorities
- Poor communication

Clinical inertia

System barriers
- Time constraints
- Work load pressure
- Non-specialist role of primary care providers
- Prescription restrictions
- Costs

Provider barriers
- Failure to initiate treatment
- Failure to intensify treatment
- Failure to identify comorbid conditions
- 'Wait for failure' approach
- Poor communication
- Confusion over range of treatments available
- Complexity of prescribing regimens
- Variations between guidelines

the only difference being the time frame in which the adverse event occurs: inappropriate use or misuse of a therapy leading to adverse events in minutes to hours (but may also be much longer, e.g. kidney damage from lithium treatment) and clinical inertia in years to decades (O'Connor et al., 2005). There also appears to be a greater acceptance of clinical inertia by healthcare providers (where the problem is a lack of appropriate prescription) compared with administering inappropriate medication (Strain et al., 2014).

Given that only around 41% of people in the United Kingdom are simultaneously achieving glucose, blood pressure and serum cholesterol targets (National Diabetes Audit, 2014/2015), the danger of clinical inertia is only too apparent. Retrospective cohort data for over 100,000 people with type 2 diabetes extracted from the UK Clinical Practice Research Datalink (CPRD), which is representative of the UK general population, illustrate the increased risk of cardiovascular events when treatment intensification is delayed (Paul et al., 2015). Compared to patients with an HbA1c <7% (<53 mmol/mol), higher levels of HbA1c combined with a 1-year delay in receiving treatment intensification were associated with significantly increased risks of myocardial infarction (67%), stroke (51%), heart failure (64%) and composite cardiovascular endpoints (62%).

Provider barriers

One of the problems in the management of type 2 diabetes is that the adverse event being prevented is invisible, whereas the side effects of treatment are not. Patients may be unwilling to accept therapies that cause hypoglycaemia or weight gain or that require injection, and physicians may therefore adopt a "wait for failure" approach, in the belief that non-intensification is better for the patient than potential side effects of treatment and/or limitations to lifestyle. Given the large group of drug classes that are now available to personalise treatment to overcome these problems, this can no longer be used as an excuse for withholding appropriate therapies for patients. The result of clinical inertia is that many people experience prolonged periods of poor glycaemic control. A recent retrospective study using data from the UK CPRD database for more than 80,000 people with type 2 diabetes found that time to treatment intensification has not significantly improved since the 1990s despite the wide range of treatment options available today (Khunti et al., 2013). The highest proportion of people with clinical inertia was for insulin initiation in people taking three oral anti-diabetes agents with patients remaining in poor glycaemic control for >7 years before intensification.

Additional factors that complicate the management of type 2 diabetes include the often non-specialist role of primary care providers, the range of treatment options available, the multiple dual or triple therapy options for treatment intensification and complexity of multi-drug regimens, variations in recommendations between international guidelines and the range of other concomitant diseases that must be managed simultaneously in many patients. With the increasing drive to personalise management, physicians may also be less clear about which goals they should be aiming for and in which patients. Guideline recommendations to personalise goals provide no clear recommendations on how they should be established.

Patient barriers

A number of factors within the patient's control may also influence clinical inertia, including a limited understanding of the seriousness of type 2 diabetes, non-adherence to lifestyle modifications and prescribed drug treatments, failure to attend appointments, conflicting priorities such as work commitments and health beliefs.

System barriers

Frequently reported system barriers relating to clinical inertia include the time constraints and workload pressure placed on providers, for example, in relation to the length and frequency of appointments. The time available to providers will also influence their ability to increase their own levels of knowledge and expertise, keep up to date with changing recommendations and new treatments, and interpret and implement evidence from clinical trials. Further system-level barriers may include local prescribing restrictions based on cost and the trend for shifting chronic disease management from secondary to primary care (Zafar et al., 2015).

OVERCOMING CLINICAL INERTIA

Given that time to treatment intensification has improved little in the past 25 years despite the wide range of varied treatments now available, new strategies are required to overcome clinical inertia. Studies in hypertension suggest that clinical inertia is more common when there is clinical uncertainty over whether action is needed (Phillips and Twombly, 2008). This may explain why it is seen more often within complex clinical situations, for example, in patients with comorbidities on a number of concomitant medications, and in older and frail patients. Some aspects of clinical inertia may therefore be a result of conflicting or unaddressed issues in the management of the disease and in the applicability of guidelines to specific groups of patients in whom evidence is lacking (Aujoulat et al., 2014). Providers should pay particular attention to these groups when evaluating type 2 diabetes management. For example, when treating older people with type 2 diabetes, reference should be made to the International Diabetes Federation guidelines, which are specifically targeted at different groups of elderly subjects including those in care homes and receiving end-of-life care (IDF, 2013).

Most clinical practice guidelines are written on the basis that everybody has a single disease problem, with little accounting for age. In reality, especially with an ageing population, people have multiple physical and psychological comorbidities, as well as social and cultural issues that make the application of single disease recommendations more difficult.

Attempts have been made to provide clinical guidance in a form that is more user-friendly and specific to individuals, for instance, in the form of computer-assisted decision support tools or personalised therapy algorithms (Vigersky et al., 2007;

Virkamäki and Saltevo, 2011; Finnish guidelines, 2013). The most recent, developed by a group of Italian diabetologists, is an online tool consisting of six personalised therapy algorithms for type 2 diabetes based on the following clinical features: HbA1c $\geq 9\%$ or $<9\%$ (75 mmol/mol), body mass index ≥ 30 or <30 kg/m^2, occupational risk potentially related to hypoglycaemia, chronic renal failure and frail elderly status (Ceriello et al., 2014). Through self-monitoring of blood glucose, patients are phenotyped according to the occurrence of fasting/pre-prandial or post-prandial hyperglycaemia. In each of these six algorithms, the gradual choice of treatment is related to the identified phenotype.

Although algorithms such as this cannot cover all of the possible combinations encountered in daily clinical practice and do not address the concomitant diseases that a patient may have, they may help to counteract some forms of clinical inertia. An international survey of over 450 physicians to gauge opinion on the guidance showed widespread agreement ($>90\%$) on the value of the algorithms proposed, even if they did not cover all possible scenarios of people with type 2 diabetes (Gallo et al., 2015). Accessible and easy-to-use personalised algorithms may help optimise therapeutic responses while simultaneously improving tolerability and compliance, but will need to be adapted to the therapeutic options available and prescribing restrictions in place in the country of use.

Clinical inertia may also be addressed by improving communication about the disease and its management between physicians and people with type 2 diabetes (Strain et al., 2014). This is particularly important in patients who are unable to achieve agreed glycaemic targets. A recent survey of people with diabetes and treating physicians across six countries found that people had only a basic understanding of the risks of complications and the importance of good glycaemic control (Strain et al., 2014). Only a small proportion believed that lifestyle changes were important and the majority did not intend to comply. The nature of the disease and the goals of treatment must be explained in a manner that is understandable to all.

Shared decision-making requires physicians and patients to form a partnership that incorporates physicians' expertise with the patients' needs and preferences. Patients who make informed, shared decisions concerning their management are more likely to adhere to any given regime. Taking daily medication is largely in the domain of the patient, but healthcare professionals can significantly influence this by their skills in communicating and motivating patients to adopt health-improving behaviours, attend clinic visits and take their medication as prescribed. Frequent review and adjustment of therapy is then seen as a part of good diabetes care rather than a sign of treatment failure. Communication is also important to identify patients' values and priorities as these will differ significantly between individuals. For example, a small study of older people with type 2 diabetes found that almost half ranked maintaining independence as their most important outcome, whereas just over one-quarter ranked staying alive highest (Laiteerapong et al., 2011). Rather than focusing purely on glycaemic control, this approach also focuses on quality of life and maintenance of function.

Adherence to medication is also influenced by the complexity of the drug regimen prescribed. A large, retrospective cohort study has found that non-adherence was 21% less likely in individuals receiving fixed-dose combinations of oral anti-diabetes drugs than those receiving separate tablets for each drug (Lokhandwala et al., 2015). Wherever possible, consideration should therefore be given to the prescription of extended-release formulations or single tablet combinations.

Cost implications are inevitable in attempts to overcome clinical inertia, but it is anticipated that these would be more than offset in the long term by the reduction in rates of complications.

REFERENCES

Ajala O, English P, Pinkney J. Systematic review and meta-analysis of different dietary approaches to the management of type 2 diabetes. *Am J Clin Nutr* 2013;97:505–516.

Aujoulat I, Jacquemin P, Rietzschel E, Scheen A, Tréfois P, Wens J, Darras E, Hermans MP. Factors associated with clinical inertia: An integrative review. *Adv Med Educ Pract* 2014;5:141–147.

Ceriello A, Gallo M, Candido R, De Micheli A, Esposito K, Gentile S, Medea G. Personalized therapy algorithms for type 2 diabetes: A phenotype-based approach. *Pharmgenomics Pers Med* 2014;7:129–136.

Diabetes treatment algorithm from the diabetes current care guideline; 2013. Working group set up by the Finnish Medical Society Duodecim and the Finnish Society of Internal Medicine. Available from: http://www.terveysportti.fi/xmedia/ccs/varhainen_diabetes_en.html. Last accessed November 9, 2015.

Gallo M, Mannucci E, De Cosmo S, Gentile S, Candido R, De Micheli A, Di Benedetto A, Esposito K, Genovese S, Medea G, Ceriello A. Algorithms for personalized therapy of type 2 diabetes: Results of a web-based international survey. *BMJ Open Diabetes Res Care* 2015;3(1):e000109.

International Diabetes Federation. Managing older people with type 2 diabetes. Global guideline; 2013. Available from: http://www.idf.org/sites/default/files/IDF-Guideline-for-older-people-T2D.pdf. Last accessed November 2015.

Khunti K, Wolden ML, Thorsted BL, Andersen M, Davies MJ. Clinical inertia in people with type 2 diabetes: A retrospective cohort study of more than 80,000 people. *Diabetes Care* 2013;36:3411–3417.

Laiteerapong N, Huang ES, Chin MH. Prioritization of care in adults with diabetes and comorbidity. *Ann N Y Acad Sci* 2011;1243:69–87.

Liebl A, Khunti K, Orozco-Beltran D, Yale JF. Health economic evaluation of type 2 diabetes mellitus: A clinical practice focused review. *Clin Med Insights Endocrinol Diabetes* 2015;8:13–19.

Lokhandwala T, Smith N, Sternhufvud C, Sörstadius E, Lee WC, Mukherjee J. A retrospective study of persistence, adherence, and health economic outcomes of fixed-dose combination vs loose-dose combination of oral anti-diabetes drugs. *J Med Econ* 2016;19:203–212.

National Diabetes Audit—2013–2014 and 2014–2015: Report 1, Care processes and treatment targets. Available from: http://www.hscic.gov.uk/catalogue/PUB19900/nati-diab-rep1-audi-2013-15.pdf. Last accessed February 2016.

National Institute for Health and Care Excellence. Type 2 diabetes in adults: management. Clinical Guideline Update (NG28). Methods, evidence and recommendations, December 2015. Available from: https://www.nice.org.uk/guidance/ng28. Last accessed 1 March 2016.

O'Connor PJ, Sperl-Hillen JM, Johnson PE, Rush WA, Biltz G. Clinical inertia and outpatient medical errors. Advances in patient safety. In: Henriksen K, Battles JB, Marks ES, Lewin DI, editors. *Advances in patient safety: From research to implementation* (Concepts and methodology; vol. 2). Rockville, Maryland): Agency for Healthcare Research and Quality (US); 2005 Feb; pp. 293–308.

Paul SK, Klein K, Thorsted BL, Wolden ML, Khunti K. Delay in treatment intensification increases the risks of cardiovascular events in patients with type 2 diabetes. *Cardiovasc Diabetol* 2015;14:100.

Phillips LS, Twombly JG. It's time to overcome clinical inertia. *Ann Intern Med* 2008;148:783–785.

Stone MA, Charpentier G, Doggen K, Kuss O, Lindblad U, Kellner C, Nolan J, Pazderska A, Rutten G, Trento M, Khunti K; GUIDANCE Study Group. Quality of care of people with type 2 diabetes in eight European countries: Findings from the Guideline Adherence to Enhance Care (GUIDANCE) study. *Diabetes Care* 2013;36:2628–2638.

Strain WD, Blüher M, Paldánius P. Clinical inertia in individualising care for diabetes: Is there time to do more in type 2 diabetes? *Diabetes Ther* 2014;5:347–354.

Vigersky RA, Galen RS, Horne D, Cavotta M, Rodbard D. Computer assisted decision support (CADS) for primary care of diabetes. *Telemed E-Health* 2007;13:168.

Virkamäki A, Saltevo J. Finnish current care guideline for diabetes: Interactive approach to improve individualised treatment. *Diabetologia* 2011;54:1264–1265.

Zafar A, Stone MA, Davies MJ, Khunti K. Acknowledging and allocating responsibility for clinical inertia in the management of Type 2 diabetes in primary care: A qualitative study. *Diabet Med* 2015;32:407–413.

3

Barriers to adherence and their solutions

Management plans in type 2 diabetes may have many components, which may be extremely challenging. These include dietary and physical activity recommendations, administration of anti-diabetes medications, self-monitoring of blood glucose, foot and eye care, and regular attendance at clinic visits. Add to this the challenges arising from other medications the patient may be receiving for other comorbid conditions, all of which have their own prescribing requirements, as well as tolerability profiles for all prescribed agents, including the potential for drug interactions. In a U.S. survey of older adults with diabetes, 50% reported using at least seven medications in their prescribed treatment regimen, including at least two glucose-lowering agents (Piette et al., 2004). Given all the above factors, it is not too surprising that adherence to management plans is one of the greatest challenges to good diabetes management. Adherence may also vary between different components of the treatment regimen so that each must be considered separately. For example, people may be adherent with their medication (anti-diabetes medication, statin), believing that this means they do not have to be adherent with their diet. In its report on adherence to long-term therapies, the World Health Organization (WHO) reported that 52%–70% of U.S. adults with type 2 diabetes adhere to diet, 26%–52% follow a physical activity plan and only about 33% self-monitor blood glucose as often as recommended (Karkashian and Schlundt, 2003).

Non-adherence to disease management regimens is widely recognized as one of the major limitations to improving healthcare outcomes (Karkashian and Schlundt, 2003). It may be intentional or non-intentional (Table 3.1) and can present in a number of different forms (Table 3.2). For example, is it because the patient is intentionally disregarding recommendations, or is he or she unable to follow them for some reason? Is there a desire on the part of the patient, but some sort of barrier that precludes adherence?

Regardless of the type of non-adherence, the consequences can be severe. Decreasing levels of adherence are consistently associated with smaller reductions in HbA1c (Farmer et al., 2016). An analysis of data from UK general practice records, which adjusted for confounding factors such as age, sex, clinical values (body mass index, HbA1c, cholesterol and blood pressure), smoking status and morbidity, found that medication non-adherence and clinic non-attendance were independent risk factors for all-cause mortality in people with type 2 diabetes (Currie et al., 2012). Misjudgement of patient adherence can also result in withholding therapy or unnecessary changes in therapy. As a consequence, reduced adherence may not only result in poor health outcomes

Table 3.1 Reasons for non-adherence: Unintentional versus intentional

Unintentional	Intentional
Forgetfulness	Mistrust
Lack of knowledge	Fear:
Poor recall of instructions	side effects (actual or perceived)
Psychiatric illness	medication is dangerous
Confusion	drug dependency
Shift work	drug–drug interactions
Work restrictions	disease stigmatization
	Lack of motivation
	No perceived benefit
	Reminder of illness
	Cost

Table 3.2 Types of non-adherence

- Receiving a prescription but not filling it
- Taking an incorrect dose
- Taking medication at the wrong times
- Increasing/decreasing the frequency of doses
- Stopping the treatment too soon
- Delay in seeking health care
- Non-participation in clinic visits
- Failure to follow doctor's instructions
- 'Drug holidays', stopping therapy for a while and then restarting
- 'White-coat compliance', only adherent to regimen around the time of clinic visits

but can also have a significant impact on healthcare costs. The overall management of type 2 diabetes should therefore address adherence as well as appropriate medications.

The majority of diabetes is self-managed with individuals providing around 95% of their own care. However, self-management can be difficult and frustrating for both patients and practitioners, particularly when there is lack of glycaemic control and continued disease progression. It is therefore important for healthcare providers to try and identify which barriers present the greatest obstacles for which patients in terms of their ability to follow the recommended disease management regimen. Once people who are non-adherent and their specific barriers have been identified, the physician can decide on which aspects of diabetes and its management to focus and can tailor adherence interventions to the needs of the individual.

WHICH PATIENTS ARE MOST AT RISK OF NON-ADHERENCE?

Barriers to adherence differ among individuals and can vary over time, but a decline in adherence is most rapid in the first 6 months after starting therapy (Osterberg and Blaschke, 2005). Sometimes, a person's non-adherence is apparent when he or she returns for a clinic visit because his or her condition has worsened or failed to improve. Others may fail to schedule or to keep appointments or fail to fill or take prescriptions as prescribed. Sometimes, non-adherence may only be discovered by careful monitoring and questioning. Healthcare providers should have a high index of suspicion for non-adherence if any of the above scenarios are regularly observed. In addition, individuals falling into one or more of the categories below may also have a higher risk of non-adherence.

Age-related morbidities

Poor adherence to prescribed regimens can affect all age groups, but older people with type 2 diabetes may be particularly at risk. They may have problems with vision, hearing and memory. It may be more difficult for them to follow therapy instructions due to cognitive impairment or other physical difficulties, such as problems swallowing tablets, opening drug containers, handling small tablets, distinguishing colours or identifying markings on drugs. Age-related alterations in pharmacokinetics and pharmacodynamics and multiple comorbidities and complex medical regimens make this population even more vulnerable to problems resulting from non-adherence. However, most cases of non-adherence in older individuals are likely to be non-intentional, and with help and support from healthcare providers or family members, adherence can be improved.

Lifestyle challenges

People may find it difficult to integrate treatment recommendations and lifestyle interventions into their schedule of daily activity because of work and other commitments. When people are too busy with their work–life schedule, they are more likely to eat unhealthily, skip meals or eat at irregular times, which may result in missing or delaying medication doses. Employment that takes people away from home and shift work also affects adherence, making it harder to follow diet and lifestyle interventions and take medication as prescribed.

Change in situation

The stress of a changing situation such as separation, divorce, death of a family member or unemployment may cause some people to temporarily adopt unhealthy self-management habits. In these situations, people who have emotional support and help from family members, friends or healthcare providers to encourage diet and exercise behaviours, and facilitate adherence with medication are more likely to be adherent.

Loss or lack of motivation

People may find it difficult to become motivated following a diagnosis of type 2 diabetes, particularly when they are asymptomatic even without strict adherence to the treatment regimen and cannot visualize the benefits of long-term therapy. It may take months or years for newly diagnosed individuals to come to terms with the serious health threat posed by diabetes (O'Connor et al., 1997). In this respect, healthcare professionals have a vital role in providing a positive attitude to what needs to be/can be done, but also sensitively imparting information that this is a condition which needs to be taken seriously even if the patient presently feels well. Unfortunately, it is often deteriorating health or major life events that are the impetus for people to make significant lifestyle changes. For others, a lack of motivation may develop over time, for example, in the absence of significant improvements in glycaemic control despite all their efforts to the contrary.

A U.S. survey of people with type 2 diabetes that explored barriers to self-management found that a moderate diet was seen as a greater burden than oral anti-diabetes agents, but less of a burden than insulin, whereas a strict diet aimed at weight loss was rated as being similarly burdensome to insulin (Vijan et al., 2005). Our modern environment can make it difficult to maintain a healthy diet. Inexpensive fast foods high in fat, salt and calories are available everywhere and are heavily marketed so that bad food habits are formed at an early age. At the same time, there is less opportunity for physical activity. Many of us drive to work, sit at a desk or stand at a counter all day, drive home and then relax in front of the television. Although these environmental risk factors are modifiable, they require significant encouragement from the healthcare provider and motivation on the side of the affected individual to look ahead, rather than just focus on short-term achievements such as reducing blood glucose levels.

Depression

The incidence of depression in type 2 diabetes is double that seen in the general population (Anderson et al., 2001) and may negatively affect how individuals take care of themselves. The depression-related symptoms such as loss of interest, impaired decision making ability and fatigue reduce the ability of people with diabetes to manage their condition, which can result in poorer control of blood glucose and difficulty in sticking to exercise, diet and treatment programmes (Egede and Ellis, 2008). Thus starts a vicious circle whereby depression may deteriorate blood glucose control through impaired self-management practices, and poor glycaemic control may aggravate depressive symptoms.

Ethnicity

People from minority ethnic backgrounds often experience particular problems with understanding information about their care, particularly when English is not their first language. These problems are exacerbated by the significantly increased risk of developing type 2 diabetes in these populations (Tillin et al., 2013). Cultural differences in diet, attitude towards exercise, health and religious beliefs, and close attachment to family traditions mean that much of the available information may not be relevant. Individuals from ethnic minorities may also be subject to social inequalities.

Poor perception and knowledge of disease

Most non-adherence is thought to be intentional in that patients make rational decisions not to take the medicine as prescribed based on their knowledge and values. For example, some patients may deny that they are ill. A prescribed medication regimen can therefore only serve as an unwelcome reminder, and the patient is unlikely to adhere to it. Others may have been frightened or confused by media reports around a drug that was once considered safe, but is now associated with health warnings or has even been withdrawn from the market.

Health literacy, defined as the ability to read, understand and remember medication instructions and act on health information (Vlasnik et al., 2005), is also important as it is difficult for patients to take a medicine when they do not understand why it is prescribed, what conditions or diseases it treats or what it prevents.

Problems with therapy

Drug therapy to control blood glucose and associated conditions can only be effective with adherence to the overall prescribed regimen. A number of therapy-related factors can affect adherence, including those associated with the complexity of the dosing regimen, frequent changes in treatment, the immediacy of beneficial effects, fear of injections and/or a therapy, and safety and most importantly tolerability.

COMPLEXITY OF DOSING REGIMEN

The chronic progressive nature of type 2 diabetes means that the complexity of the medication regimen is likely to increase over time. In general, adherence with oral anti-diabetes agents declines as the number of drugs increases (Mateo et al., 2006). Adherence is also inversely proportional to the number of times a day medication must be taken (Claxton et al., 2012). For medication taken only once daily, the average adherence rate is nearly 80%; for medication that must be taken 4 times a day, the average rate drops to about 50%. However, even an adherence rate of 80% means missing one of every five doses of a once-daily medication, or one to two doses per week.

For people struggling with the complexity of a dosing regimen, modifications may involve decreasing the number of therapies and frequency of therapy, and altering the route of administration. There are a number of fixed-dose combinations with different mechanisms of action for the treatment of hyperglycaemia, which demonstrate bioequivalence to the separate tablets, but with reduced pill burden, increased patient adherence and improvements in glycaemic control (Han et al., 2012). Data from a physician interview study have also indicated that the decision to prescribe a fixed-dose combination was associated with improved treatment satisfaction among patients (Benford et al., 2012). Currently available fixed-dose combinations include metformin combined with a sulphonylurea, thiazolidinedione, dipeptidylpeptidase-4 inhibitor, glinide or sodium-glucose cotransporter-2 inhibitor, as well as thiazolidinedione–sulphonylurea combinations. These are available at a range of dosage strengths to facilitate titration.

FEAR OF INJECTIONS

Adherence to injectable regimens is lower than that to oral drugs, and many people with diabetes are reluctant to start them. Some of the barriers to injectable medications can be overcome by education and counselling, but resistance and clinical inertia remains a problem because of the lifelong nature of the disease.

Although most barriers to adherence apply to all therapies, there may be greater and/or additional barriers associated with initiating and adhering to insulin. In addition to fearing needles, many people with diabetes are keen to avoid starting insulin because they believe it signals a worsening of their disease. Other factors often cited as barriers to using insulin include pain of injection, permanence of therapy, restrictiveness and concern about hypoglycaemia and weight gain (Polonsky et al., 2005).

Some healthcare providers may worsen psychological insulin resistance by using insulin as a 'threat' if current medications fail to achieve blood glucose control. The mindset of psychological insulin resistance may be minimized by advising people early on and continually that insulin is a safe and effective medication for lowering blood glucose and might be required at some point in their lives to manage the disease. There have also been many improvements in insulin therapy to aid adherence such as the use of pen-like devices to overcome fear of conventional syringe and needles, and the availability of modern insulin analogues, including the rapid-acting analogues (aspart, lispro, glulisine), the long-acting basal analogues (glargine, detemir) and the premixed insulin analogue formulations, all of which have been developed to allow for a closer replication of a normal insulin profile.

SAFETY AND TOLERABILITY

Adverse effects, or fear of adverse effects, can be a major barrier to medication adherence, and indeed some studies have suggested that poor tolerability may be the single biggest reason for poor adherence to pharmacotherapy (Figure 3.1) (Grant et al., 2003). In particular, fear of hypoglycaemia and weight gain may discourage adherence to regimens involving insulin or insulin secretagogues (sulphonylureas and glinides).

Weight gain

A high proportion of people with type 2 diabetes are overweight or obese at diagnosis. An exploratory survey among 121 people with type 2 diabetes showed that 32.8% thought medication would cause unpleasant side effects and 13.9% thought it would lead to

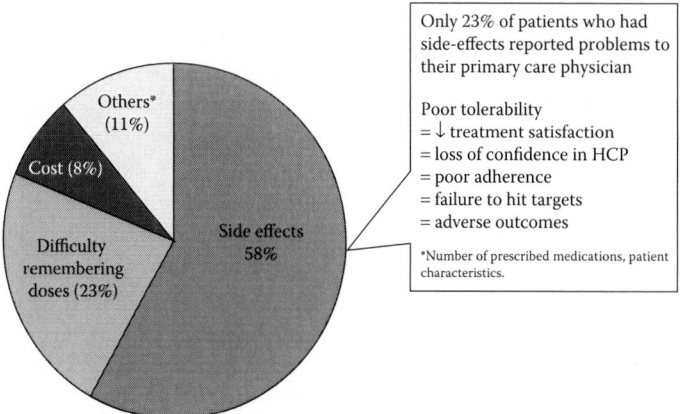

Figure 3.1 Most common factors related to non-adherence in patients with type 2 diabetes. (Grant, R.W. et al., *Diabetes Care*, 26, 1408–1412, 2003.)

weight gain, and these factors were associated with reduced medication adherence (Farmer et al., 2006). In a retrospective study of 294 people with type 2 diabetes, those who were obese or severely obese were more than twice as likely to have low or moderate adherence compared with those who were not obese (Dilla et al., 2008). A range of anti-diabetes medications are available that are either weight neutral or lead to reductions in weight.

Hypoglycaemia

The risk of hypoglycaemia is increased in insulin-treated diabetes, but is also present when diabetes is managed with insulin secretagogues alone or in combination with other agents. Other factors may increase risk such as unaccustomed or strenuous physical activity, stress, excessive alcohol consumption, acute illness or variation in normal carbohydrate intake, for example, skipping meals, can all contribute to hypoglycaemia. It is often difficult for people with diabetes to understand the relationships between the different aspects of diabetes management that can lead to hypoglycaemia.

As a result of the associated unpleasant symptoms and health risks, individuals with diabetes generally try to avoid hypoglycaemia. Fear of hypoglycaemia can be an important barrier to good diabetes self-management and may lead some to maintain high blood glucose levels to avoid it. There is now a range of anti-diabetes medications that do not cause hypoglycaemia. The risk of severe hypoglycaemia is also reduced with the rapid-acting insulin analogues compared with human soluble insulin and with the basal insulin analogues, for example, glargine and detemir, compared with neutral protamine hagedorn insulin. Blood glucose awareness training helps reduce the fear of hypoglycaemia as well as the frequency of the episodes.

Gastrointestinal problems

Metformin is the most commonly prescribed oral anti-diabetes agent used in the treatment of type 2 diabetes and is the first-line option in all treatment guidelines. However, up to 25% of patients develop gastrointestinal side effects leading to cessation in 5%–10% of users. Extended-release metformin is associated with significantly less gastrointestinal events than immediate-release metformin, and adherence has been shown to be significantly greater in patients who used this formulation compared with those who took the immediate-release medication (Donnelly et al., 2009).

Lack of knowledge

A lack of knowledge and understanding about the disease, the purpose of taking medication, and when to take the medication to get the best therapeutic effect with the fewest adverse effects is a major barrier to diabetes management. The elderly are particularly vulnerable, often having a lack of basic knowledge that increases in those with cognitive impairment.

The level of self-management required in chronic diseases such as diabetes means that there is a high need for information. However, providing generic educational materials that may not be relevant to the individual is not enough. The real challenge is how to ensure that the information has not only increased knowledge but also resulted in a behavioural change. For example, some people may need help in fitting their management around their work and/or leisure activities. Others may be reluctant to adjust their insulin dose because they are afraid of making mistakes, which could lead to hypoglycaemia. The aim of patient education for people with diabetes is to improve their knowledge, skills and confidence, enabling them to take increasing control of their condition and integrate effective and safe self-management into their daily lives.

A meta-analysis of studies that tested interventions to improve diabetes self-management found that combining behavioural techniques with provision of information was more effective than interventions that provided information alone (Brown, 1999). This need to actively involve individuals with type 2 diabetes in the learning process was the basis for the development of diabetes self-management education initiatives such as Diabetes Education and Self-Management for Ongoing and Newly Diagnosed (DESMOND), which help people gain the knowledge and skills necessary to modify their behaviour and successfully manage the disease.

The DESMOND philosophy recognizes that personalising health risks may improve motivation. The series of self-management education workshops provide individuals with only basic information from which to learn (Davies et al., 2008). For example, the workshop might use the analogy that having insulin resistance is similar to having a rusty lock on your front door. Insulin is the key that unlocks the door, but because it is rusty, the lock in the door is not working well. Facilitators then support individuals to work out how this information relates to what is happening in their bodies now and in the future (e.g. that because they are resistant to insulin, their pancreas needs to work harder and may then get tired out and start being inefficient) (Skinner et al., 2003). This helps individuals understand how the information relates to what is happening in their own bodies and is therefore more likely to be retained. In all DESMOND modules, individuals are supported to identify their own health risks and then respond by setting personalised goals that are behavioural and specific. Importantly, there are also specific workshops for ethnic minority groups.

HOW TO QUESTION PATIENTS ABOUT NON-ADHERENCE

A common challenge faced by a healthcare professional is whether a patient's elevated levels of blood glucose are due to poor adherence or progression of the disease despite proper medication. Questioning around the predictive factors for non-adherence described in this chapter may help provide the answers.

People are more likely to confide their fears of side effects and other barriers to self-management if they have a long-standing, trusting relationship with their healthcare professional. A healthy relationship is based on patients' trust in physicians and other relevant professionals and empathy. Adherence is better when health care professionals are emotionally supportive, provide reassurance and treat patients as an equal partner.

How questions are phrased is important because patients generally want to please their doctor. Rather than asking a question that can be answered with a 'yes' or 'no' answer (e.g. 'Are you experiencing any problems with the medicines?'), ask how your patients are taking the medication or how many doses they think they have missed in the last week. Questioning should be specific; for example, taking medicines every day can be a real inconvenience for some people, when do you have the most difficulty keeping to your treatment plan? Ask about how/when patients are taking their medication and whether they are experiencing any of the major known side effects.

A common reaction to non-adherence is to describe what the patients' future could hold if they do not start taking their medication as prescribed. However, this can make patients feel shamed and that they have done something wrong, and in future visits, they may not reveal non-adherence for fear of the same reaction. When patients reveal non-adherence, it is important to assure them that it is a positive step that they felt comfortable telling you. Emphasize that now you can work together to identify a solution.

TAILOR ADHERENCE SOLUTION TO NON-ADHERENCE PROBLEM

Adherence interventions should be tailored to the needs of the patient (Figure 3.2, Table 3.3). In those who are asymptomatic, understanding the patient's perspective is vital. Empathic comments, such as 'It is difficult to take a medicine when you don't

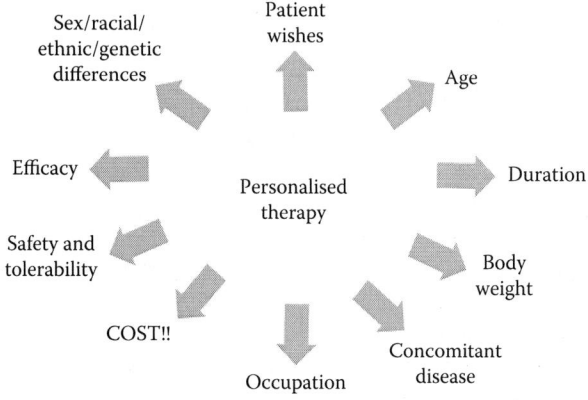

Figure 3.2 Tailored therapy in type 2 diabetes: Patient considerations.

Table 3.3 Factors associated with improved adherence to medications taken by patients with type 2 diabetes

Reduced treatment complexity, oral agents, fixed-dose combinations and decreased frequency of administration

Medications that are weight neutral or weight reducing, and with glucose-dependent effects, leading to decreased/low risk of hypoglycaemia and other side effects

Education and increased knowledge

Ensure treatment benefits outweigh costs

Good patient–healthcare provider relationship. Improved continuity of care and increased communication through websites and electronic records

Source: Adapted from García-Pérez et al., *Diabetes Ther,* 4, 175–194, 2013.

feel any different whether you take it or not', build a trusting relationship.

Taking single daily doses is far easier for patients with chronic diseases. This may involve extended-release formulations or fixed-dose combinations. People who achieve blood glucose control with few or no adverse events, such as weight gain and hypoglycaemia, are more likely to remain adherent. A number of currently available anti-diabetes medications are effective in lowering glucose without these side effects.

CONCLUSIONS

There is little doubt that poor adherence to management plans is a major (possibly the biggest) challenge to achievement of good glycaemic (and other risk factor) control in people with type 2 diabetes. There are a multiplicity of factors that relate to poor adherence, and undoubtedly, some of these can be mitigated if appropriate steps are taken.

Personalised care will not only reduce the risk of clinical inertia as discussed in Chapter 2, but is also critical in supporting patients to improve adherence. From a pharmacotherapeutic perspective, this can involve, for example, discussing with patients the pros and cons of various therapies, avoidance where possible of drugs which cause weight gain and hypoglycaemia, use of fixed-dose combinations where appropriate to reduce tablet load, and all this aided by good multi-professional support and educational programmes. The patient must be the central player in the organisation of his or her management plan. In this way, patients are much more likely to 'buy in to' what will be required of them in order to sustain a healthy life and reduce the risks of long-term complications.

REFERENCES

Anderson RJ, Freedland KE, Clouse RE, Lustman PJ. The prevalence of comorbid depression in adults with diabetes: A meta-analysis. *Diabetes Care* 2001;24:1069–1078.

Benford M, Milligan G, Pike J, Anderson P, Piercy J, Fermer S. Fixed-dose combination antidiabetic therapy: Real-world factors associated with prescribing choices and relationship with patient satisfaction and compliance. *Adv Ther* 2012;29:26–40.

Brown SA. Interventions to promote diabetes self-management: State of the science. *Diabetes Educ* 1999;25:52–61.

Claxton AJ, Cramer J, Pierce C. A systematic review of the associations between dose regimens and medication compliance. *Clin Ther* 2012;23:1296–1310.

Currie CJ, Peyrot M, Morgan CL, Poole CD, Jenkins-Jones S, Rubin RR, Burton CM, Evans M. The impact of treatment noncompliance on mortality in people with type 2 diabetes. *Diabetes Care* 2012;35:1279–1284.

Davies MJ, Heller S, Skinner TC et al.; Diabetes Education and Self Management for Ongoing and Newly Diagnosed Collaborative. Effectiveness of the diabetes education and self management for ongoing and newly diagnosed (DESMOND) programme for people with newly diagnosed type 2 diabetes: Cluster randomised controlled trial. *BMJ* 2008;336:491–495.

Dilla T, Costi M, Boye KS et al. The impact of obesity in the management and evolution of diabetes mellitus. *Rev Clin Esp* 2008;208:437–443.

Donnelly LA, Morris AD, Pearson ER. Adherence in patients transferred from immediate release metformin to a sustained release formulation: A population-based study. *Diabetes Obes Metab* 2009;11:338–342.

Egede LE, Ellis C. The effects of depression on diabetes knowledge, diabetes self-management, and perceived control in indigent patients with type 2 diabetes. *Diabetes Technol Ther* 2008;10:213–219.

Farmer A, Kinmonth AL, Sutton S. Measuring beliefs about taking hypoglycaemic medication among people with type 2 diabetes. *Diabet Med* 2006;23:265–270.

Farmer AJ, Rodgers LR, Lonergan M et al.; MASTERMIND Consortium. Adherence to oral glucose-lowering therapies and associations with 1-year HbA1c: A retrospective cohort analysis in a large primary care database. *Diabetes Care* 2016;39:258–263.

García-Pérez L-E, Alvarez M, Dilla T, Gil-Guillén V, Orozco-Beltrán D. Adherence to therapies in patients with type 2 diabetes. *Diabetes Ther* 2013;4:175–194.

Grant RW, Devita NG, Singer DE, Meigs JB. Polypharmacy and medication adherence in patients with type 2 diabetes. *Diabetes Care* 2003;26:1408–1412.

Han S, Iglay K, Davies MJ, Zhang Q, Radican L. Glycemic effectiveness and medication adherence with fixed-dose combination or coadministered dual therapy of antihyperglycemic regimens: A meta-analysis. *Curr Med Res Opin* 2012;28:969–977.

Karkashian C, Schlundt D. Diabetes. In: Sabate E, ed. *Adherence to long-term therapies: Evidence for action*. Geneva, Switzerland: World Health Organization; 2003. pp. 71–85. Available from: http://www.who.int/chp/knowledge/publications/adherence_full_report.pdf. Last accessed January 24, 2016.

Mateo JF, Gil-Guillén VF, Mateo E, Orozco D, Carbayo JA, Merino J. Multifactorial approach and adherence to prescribed oral medications in patients with type 2 diabetes. *Int J Clin Pract* 2006;60:422–428.

O'Connor PJ, Crabtree BF, Yanoshik MK. Differences between diabetic patients who do and do not respond to a diabetes care intervention: A qualitative analysis. *Fam Med* 1997;29:424–428.

Osterberg L, Blaschke T. Adherence to medication. *N Engl J Med* 2005;353:487–497.

Piette JD, Heisler M, Wagner TH. Problems paying out-of-pocket medication costs among older adults with diabetes. *Diabetes Care* 2004;27:384–391.

Polonsky WH, Fisher L, Guzman S, Villa-Caballero L, Edelman SV. Psychological insulin resistance in patients with type 2 diabetes: The scope of the problem. *Diabetes Care* 2005;28:2543–2546.

Skinner TC, Cradock S, Arundel F, Graham W. Four theories and a philosophy: Self-management education for individuals newly diagnosed with type 2 diabetes. *Diabetes Spectrum* 2003;16:75–80.

Tillin T, Hughes AD, Godsland IF et al. Insulin resistance and truncal obesity as important determinants of the greater incidence of diabetes in Indian Asians and African Caribbeans compared with Europeans: The Southall And Brent REvisited (SABRE) cohort. Diabetes Care 2013;36:383–393.

Vijan S, Stuart NS, Fitzgerald JT, Ronis DL, Hayward RA, Slater S, Hofer TP. Barriers to following dietary recommendations in Type 2 diabetes. *Diabet Med* 2005;22:32–38.

Vlasnik JJ, Aliotta SL, DeLor B. Medication adherence: Factors influencing compliance with prescribed medication plans. *Case Manager* 2005;16:47–51.

4

Advantages and disadvantages of new therapies

Efficacy based on haemoglobin A1c (HbA1c) lowering and tolerability are no longer the only criteria for the success of a new drug for type 2 diabetes; ease of administration, convenient dosing, weight reductions or weight neutrality, a low hypoglycaemic risk and beneficial effects on cardiovascular outcomes are all important factors.

Type 2 diabetes is associated with a number of pathophysiological abnormalities, including peripheral insulin resistance, impaired regulation of hepatic glucose production and declining β-cell function. No single anti-diabetes agent can correct all the abnormalities. In addition, the decrease in HbA1c that can be achieved with a single agent is, at most, 1.0%–1.5% (11–16 mmol/mol) depending upon the starting level. In people with newly diagnosed type 2 diabetes and HbA1c >8.0% (64 mmol/mol), lifestyle changes and a single pharmacotherapeutic agent commonly will not achieve and maintain appropriate blood glucose levels. Options in this case are to prescribe combination therapy immediately or to intensify beyond first-line therapy promptly if glycaemic targets are not rapidly achieved (say within 3 months). The newer agents fulfil a need for treatments with mechanisms of action that can be used in combination, providing additive blood glucose control with a low risk of adverse events, such as hypoglycaemia or weight gain. For these reasons, more modern agents may have important advantages over some of the older therapies (Tahrani et al., 2016).

OLDER THERAPIES

Metformin

Metformin primarily reduces elevated blood glucose by decreasing hepatic glucose production and, to a lesser extent, by decreasing peripheral insulin resistance. It does not stimulate insulin release. There is universal agreement among guidelines for the management of type 2 diabetes for metformin as first-line therapy in those in whom lifestyle interventions are insufficient to control hyperglycaemia. In addition to achieving significant reductions in HbA1c, it does not cause weight gain or hypoglycaemia, improves lipid profiles and may have possible benefits on cardiovascular outcomes. There is also preliminary evidence that it may protect against certain types of cancer. It is one of the least expensive oral anti-diabetes agents.

Metformin is very rarely associated with lactic acidosis, and as its major route of excretion is via the kidneys, it has been contra-indicated in people with renal failure. However, since this labelling was established several decades ago, research has shown no increased risk for lactic acidosis in patients with mild to moderately impaired renal function (estimated glomerular filtration rates [eGFRs], 30–60 mL/min per 1.73 m^2) (Ekström et al., 2012; Inzucchi et al., 2014). The National Institute for Health and Care Excellence (NICE) suggests that metformin should not be started with an eGFR <45 mL/min (NICE, 2015). However, it advises if a patient is already suitably controlled using metformin, it may be appropriate to continue its use down to an eGFR of 30 mL/min, provided there is frequent monitoring of renal function and appropriate dose adjustment.

The major drawback with conventional metformin therapy is the requirement for multiple daily doses and dose escalation-related gastrointestinal side effects, although these can be reduced by appropriate titration and dosing prior to or with meals.

Modified-release metformin

A modified-release formulation of metformin has been developed, which is administered once daily and is now available generically. The slower absorption with this formulation may improve gastro-intestinal tolerability in some patients and allow for more convenient once-daily dosing which can improve adherence. NICE 2015 guidelines suggest that a trial of modified-release metformin can be initiated if a patient experiences gastrointestinal side effects with standard-release metformin (NICE, 2015).

Sulphonylureas

Sulphonylureas increase insulin secretion by binding to specific receptors on the β cells, resulting in closure of potassium ATP channels. This leads to β-cell depolarization, influx of calcium and activation of the secretory machinery that releases insulin. They require some residual β-cell function for their blood glucose-lowering effect. Follow-up of over 17,000 drug-naive people in the Swedish National Diabetes Register has shown that when used as monotherapy, sulphonylureas (and glinides) were associated with a substantially increased risk of switch to a new agent or addition of a second agent compared with metformin indicating reduced glycaemic durability (Ekström et al., 2015).

Until recently, sulphonylureas have been considered the drug of choice for add-on therapy to metformin. They vary considerably in their metabolism and route of elimination, but all are associated with weight gain and with hypoglycaemia as they stimulate insulin secretion virtually independently of plasma glucose levels. The risk is lower with shorter acting agents than those which are either long acting per se or give rise to active metabolites that substantially prolong their pharmacodynamic effects, such as glibenclamide and chlorpropamide. To avoid accumulation and increased risk of hypoglycaemia, long-acting agents should be particularly avoided in the elderly and those with renal impairment. Given the risks of hypoglycaemia with all sulphonylureas, it is the author's opinion that as far as possible sulphonylureas should be avoided in these types of high-risk patients, particularly because other agents that do not increase hypoglycaemia risk are now available.

Sulphonylureas are also listed as an option for initial therapy in patients in whom metformin is contraindicated or not tolerated and as a dual therapy option with metformin in both the latest NICE and European Association for the Study of Diabetes (EASD)/ American Diabetes Association (ADA) guidelines. They can also be particularly useful as first-line agents in patients who are significantly symptomatic at diagnosis as they work rapidly to improve glycaemic control and symptoms. Given their lack of durability and problems of weight gain and hypoglycaemia, if such an approach is used, it is the author's practice to switch to an alternative agent once management is established and symptoms improved/relieved.

Meglitinides

Meglitinides or glinides have a similar mechanism of action to the sulphonylureas, but differ in their β-cell binding sites, receptor affinity and absorption and elimination rates. This results in differences in potency, rate of onset and duration of action. The glinides are rapid-acting insulin secretagogues that lower post-prandial glucose excursions by targeting early-phase insulin release, but have no impact on fasting glucose. As with the sulphonylureas, glinide-induced insulin stimulation is dependent on functioning pancreatic β cells. Although repaglinide has been approved for almost 20 years, there have been no relevant trials to date of longer duration than 14 months and therefore no long-term outcome data. The multiple dosing requirements of repaglinide (15 min before a meal) have previously inhibited uptake in clinical practice. A meta-analysis has shown that the risk of hypoglycaemia is at least as high as that of sulphonylureas with similar weight gain (Phung et al., 2010). Finally, repaglinide is only authorised for use as monotherapy or in combination with metformin, meaning that if optimal results are not achieved as initial therapy, no licensed options to intensify with another agent are available.

Thiazolidinediones (glitazones)

These agents decrease fasting and post-prandial plasma glucose by improving the sensitivity of hepatic and peripheral (muscle) tissues to insulin and result in more sustained improvements in glycaemic control than with either metformin or (particularly) the sulphonylureas. Pioglitazone and other thiazolidinediones initially showed great promise as oral therapies for type 2 diabetes, but a host of potentially serious side effects have limited their use, including fluid retention, promotion of heart failure, bone fractures and a caution for bladder cancer. The European Medicines Agency removed rosiglitazone's marketing authorisation across Europe in 2010 because of concerns about cardiovascular safety.

Pioglitazone does not increase the risk of hypoglycaemia, but is renowned for promoting weight gain. It may still have a therapeutic role in the management of selected patients, but care should be taken, given it is associated with weight gain and oedema and an increased risk of heart failure. Fracture risk also needs to be seriously considered particularly in the elderly and specifically in postmenopausal women. It remains an option for initial therapy in patients in whom metformin is contraindicated or not tolerated and as a dual or triple therapy option with metformin in both the latest NICE and EASD/ADA guidelines.

Alpha-glucosidase inhibitors

Alpha-glucosidase inhibitors (e.g. acarbose) act by inhibiting alpha-glucosidase in the brush border cells that line the small intestine, which cleaves more complex carbohydrates into sugars. The greatest effect of this agent is therefore on post-prandial hyperglycaemia, and HbA1c reductions are in the region of 0.5% (5.5 mmol/mol). Gastrointestinal side effects are extremely common and include abdominal discomfort, bloating, flatulence and diarrhoea. Therapy with acarbose has been linked to elevations in serum transaminase levels, and the use of this agent is contraindicated in patients with liver cirrhosis. Likewise, concentrations have been shown to increase proportionally with the degree of renal dysfunction. Other contraindications include patients with inflammatory bowel disease or a history of bowel obstruction. These agents are rarely used in Europe but more commonly in China, Japan and elsewhere.

NEWER THERAPIES

Incretin-based therapies

These include the dipeptidyl peptidase-4 (DPP-4) inhibitors (gliptins) and glucagon-like peptide 1 receptor agonists (GLP-1 RAs).

Their development was based on the science behind the role of GLP-1 in glucose homeostasis. GLP-1 is a naturally occurring molecule secreted by the gut in response to food. It promotes insulin secretion from the pancreatic β cells and inhibits glucagon secretion from the pancreatic alpha cells, the latter then inhibiting hepatic glucose production. GLP-1 slows stomach emptying, provoking a feeling of 'fullness' and reducing post-prandial hyperglycaemia. It also has a central appetite suppressant effect. Importantly, GLP-1 secretion is glucose dependent; that is, it only exerts its effects in response to a meal when glucose levels are rising or high and its effect 'switches off' once glucose levels normalise.

In people with type 2 diabetes, continuous intravenous infusion of GLP-1 has a dramatic effect in improving glucose control. It is not a practical option as a therapy, however, as it has a half-life of only 1–2 min. This is because it is very rapidly broken down by the naturally occurring enzyme DPP-4 to inactive products. This has led to the development of two new drug classes: (1) the DPP-4 inhibitors that allow naturally produced GLP-1 to act for longer and (2) GLP-1 RAs that have similar actions to GLP-1 but are not broken down by DPP-4. This prolongs their active life and allows them to be given by subcutaneous injection twice daily, once daily or even once weekly depending on the characteristics of the GLP-1 RA in question.

DPP-4 inhibitors

The DPP-4 inhibitors increase GLP-1 availability by preventing its degradation. As stimulation of the GLP-1 receptor is indirect, increases in endogenous GLP-1 and decreases in glucagon secretion are more modest than with the GLP-1 RAs. DPP-4 inhibitors predominantly affect the post-prandial plasma glucose excursion, but a modest reduction in fasting plasma glucose is also observed. They are approved for treatment of hyperglycaemia as mono-, dual and triple oral therapies as well as in combination with insulin. A large meta-analysis of DPP-4 inhibitor trials reported that compared with placebo, the DPP-4 inhibitors reduced HbA1c by around 0.7% (Monami et al., 2010). The efficacy was similar in monotherapy and in combination with other agents. They are not associated with weight gain and have a very low risk of hypoglycaemia. DPP-4 inhibitors are administered once daily in tablet form (sitagliptin, saxagliptin, alogliptin, linagliptin), except vildagliptin that is given twice daily. All are also available as fixed-dose combinations with metformin, and linagliptin is also available as a fixed-dose combination with the sodium-glucose cotransporter-2 (SGLT-2) inhibitor empagliflozin.

The DPP-4 inhibitors are generally extremely well tolerated, and the most frequent adverse event in clinical trials was nasopharyngitis. Like the GLP-1 RAs, pancreatitis has been reported in post-marketing surveillance for the DPP-4 inhibitors, and their use should be avoided in patients with a history (or at high risk) of the condition. The U.S. Food and Drug Administration (FDA) has also recently added a new warning about the potential risk for severe joint pain to the labels of all products in the DPP-4 inhibitor class.

Most DPP-4 inhibitors (sitagliptin, vildagliptin, saxagliptin, alogliptin) are predominantly cleared by renal excretion, but with differences in active metabolites. As a result, the total exposure to the drug is increased in proportion to the decline of GFR, leading to recommendations for appropriate dose reductions according to the severity of chronic kidney disease (CKD). Sitagliptin is largely excreted unchanged in the urine, but can be used with dose reduction. Vildagliptin is metabolised to inactive metabolites, which are then renally excreted. Usually given at a dose of 50 mg twice daily, this should be halved to 50 mg once daily in patients with moderate or severe renal impairment, and it can be used with caution in those with end-stage renal disease. Saxagliptin is metabolized mainly in the liver to an active metabolite that is renally excreted. The usual dose should be halved in patients with moderate or severe renal impairment. Linagliptin is excreted almost entirely unchanged in bile and not by renal excretion, making it a useful drug for patients with any degree of renal impairment (including dialysis) without dose adjustment.

Three cardiovascular outcome trials with the DPP-4 inhibitors have been completed. In Saxagliptin Assessment of Vascular Outcomes Recorded in Patients with Diabetes Mellitus—Thrombolysis in Myocardial Infarction 53 (SAVOR-TIMI 53) (Scirica et al., 2013) and Examination of Cardiovascular Outcomes with Alogliptin versus Standard of Care (EXAMINE) (White et al., 2013), neither saxagliptin or alogliptin differed from placebo in terms of the composite primary endpoint: cardiovascular death, non-fatal myocardial infarction (MI), and non-fatal stroke. However, in both trials, concerns were raised about heart failure. In SAVOR-TIMI 53, saxagliptin-treated subjects had significantly higher rates of heart failure hospitalisation (but not heart failure-related mortality) compared with placebo: 3.5% ($n = 289$) vs. 2.8% ($n = 228$) over 2.1 years of follow-up (hazard ratio [HR] 1.27; 95% confidence interval [CI] 1.07–1.51; $p = .007$). Post-hoc analyses of the EXAMINE trial showed that, over a relatively short follow-up of 1.5 years, hospitalisation for heart failure occurred in numerically more patients receiving alogliptin than placebo (3.9% [$n = 106$] vs. 3.3% [$n = 89$]; HR 1.19; 95% CI 0.90–1.58; $p = .22$), but this was not significant.

The Trial Evaluating Cardiovascular Outcomes with Sitagliptin (TECOS) randomized 14,671 patients with type 2 diabetes and established cardiovascular disease to add either sitagliptin or placebo to their existing therapy (Green et al., 2015). After a median follow-up of 3.0 years, there was no difference in the primary outcome (cardiovascular death, non-fatal MI, non-fatal stroke or unstable angina) compared with placebo. Importantly, sitagliptin in the TECOS was not associated with any signal for heart failure.

Overall, the TECOS, SAVOR-TIMI 53 and EXAMINE trials have demonstrated the cardiovascular safety of the DDP-4 inhibitors in high-cardiovascular-risk patients with type 2 diabetes. A recent large observational study involving almost 1.5 million people with type 2 diabetes in the United States, Canada and the United Kingdom found that the use of incretin-based therapy was not associated with an excess risk for heart failure-related hospitalisation compared with use of other anti-diabetes drug combinations (Filion et al., 2016). This was the case for both DPP-4 inhibitors and GLP-1 RAs, and for people with and without histories of heart failure. It remains to be seen whether there are any differences between the various agents in terms of associated risk for heart failure.

In the NICE and ADA/EASD 2015 guidelines, DPP-4 inhibitors can be considered for dual therapy with metformin if blood glucose levels are not controlled on metformin monotherapy. They can also be used in combination with pioglitazone or a sulphonylurea if metformin is contraindicated or not tolerated and as a triple oral therapy option with metformin and either pioglitazone or a sulphonylurea. They can also be used as a first-line therapy where metformin is not tolerated or contraindicated.

Potential users of DPP-4 inhibitors

Because of their excellent tolerability and good safety profile, they can be used right across the spectrum of patients with type 2 diabetes and are particularly useful in the elderly, people with renal impairment (very low risk of hypoglycaemia) and where post-prandial hyperglycaemia is a significant issue.

GLP-1 receptor agonists

GLP-1 RAs provide pharmacological levels of GLP-1, activating GLP-1 receptors in the pancreas and mimicking the actions of endogenous GLP-1: glucose-dependent increase in insulin release and decrease in glucagon release with a consequent low risk for hypoglycaemia. These agents are also associated with weight reduction by their effects on delaying gastric emptying and increasing satiety.

There are currently six GLP-1 RAs approved for use in the European Union, which can be classified as short-acting (exenatide twice daily, lixisenatide once daily) or long-acting (liraglutide once daily, exenatide once weekly, albiglutide once weekly and dulaglutide once weekly) (Table 4.1). All of the GLP-1 RAs are administered as subcutaneous injections and are available as prefilled injection pens.

To date, nine phase III head-to-head trials and one large phase II study have compared the efficacy and safety of these drugs (Madsbad, 2016). All trials were associated with HbA1c reductions of between 0.8% (9 mmol/mol) and 1.9% (21 mmol/mol). In general, longer acting GLP-1 RAs (which include liraglutide despite the fact it is licensed only for once daily use) lower HbA1c to a greater extent. Exenatide twice daily partially restores the first-phase insulin response, and injections should be administered within the 60-min window PRIOR TO eating the two main meals of the day. Lixisenatide should also be given prior to the main meal of the day. The other GLP-1 RAs can be administered at any time of the day with or without meals.

In addition to improved coverage of post-prandial hyperglycaemia, the short-acting GLP-1 RAs offer greater weight reductions. The potential advantages of long-acting GLP-1 RAs include a greater action on fasting plasma glucose, less frequent injections and lower rates of nausea (Table 4.1).

GLP-1 receptors are also expressed in the heart and vasculature, and preclinical studies with GLP-1 RAs indicate that they have favourable effects on endothelial function, recovery from ischaemic injury and myocardial function (Chilton, 2015). In the first cardiovascular outcome trial to be reported with a GLP-1 RA (Evaluation of Lixisenatide in Acute Coronary Syndrome [ELIXA]), there was no increased cardiac risk (cardiovascular death, MI, stroke, unstable angina or heart failure) for lixisenatide compared with placebo in over 6000 people with type 2 diabetes who had recently experienced acute coronary syndrome events (Pfeffer et al., 2015).

The Liraglutide Effect and Action in Diabetes: Evaluation of Cardiovascular Outcome Results (LEADER) trial, which was launched in 2010 to meet FDA requirements for post-marketing cardiovascular analysis of new diabetes therapies, has also recently completed (Marso et al., 2016a). This double-blind trial randomized

Table 4.1 Comparison of GLP-1 RAs

Parameters	Short-acting GLP-1 RAs	Long-acting GLP-1 RAs
Compounds	Exenatide Lixisenatide	Albiglutide Dulaglutide Exenatide-LAR Liraglutide
Half-life	2–5 h	12 h to several days
Effects		
Fasting blood glucose levels	Modest reduction	Strong reduction
Post-prandial hyperglycaemia	Strong reduction	Modest reduction
Fasting insulin secretion	Modest stimulation	Strong stimulation
Post-prandial insulin secretion	Strong stimulation	Modest stimulation
Glucagon secretion	Reduction	Reduction
Gastric emptying rate	Deceleration	No effect
Blood pressure	Reduction	Reduction
Heart rate	No effect or small increase (0–2 bpm)	Moderate increase (2–5 bpm)
Body weight reduction	1–5 kg	2–5 kg
Induction of nausea	20%–50%, attenuates slowly (weeks to many months)	20%–40%, attenuates quickly (~4–8 weeks)

Source: Reproduced with permission from Meier, J.J., *Nature Rev Endocrinol*, 8, 728–742, 2012.
GLP-1, glucagon-like peptide 1; LAR, long-acting release.

9340 patients with type 2 diabetes at high risk of major adverse cardiovascular events to either 1.8 mg of liraglutide or placebo in addition to standard care. The primary composite outcome in the time-to-event analysis was the first occurrence of death from cardiovascular causes, non-fatal MI or non-fatal stroke. The average duration of disease was 12.9 years for placebo and 12.8 years for the liraglutide arm, and patients had a mean HbA1c of 8.7% (71.6 mmol/mol). Patients were followed for a median of 3.8 years. In addition to meeting the primary endpoint of non-inferiority, the trial also demonstrated superiority. There was a statistically significant reduction in cardiovascular risk for the liraglutide arm compared with placebo: 608 out of 4668 (13%) in the liraglutide arm and 694 of 4672 (14.9%) in the placebo arm; HR (95% CI), 0.87 (0.78–0.97); $p < .001$ for non-inferiority, $p = .01$ for superiority (Figure 4.1). Fewer patients died from cardiovascular causes in the liraglutide group (219 patients, or 4.7%) than in the placebo group (278 patients, or 6.0%) (HR [95% CI], 0.78 [0.66–0.93]; p = .007) and

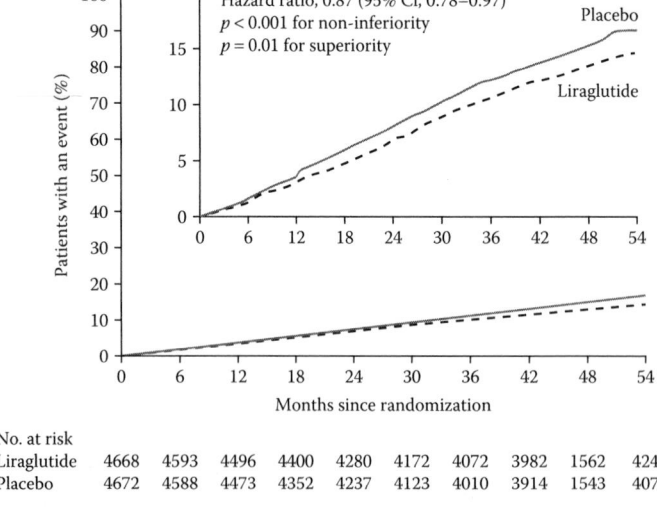

No. at risk										
Liraglutide	4668	4593	4496	4400	4280	4172	4072	3982	1562	424
Placebo	4672	4588	4473	4352	4237	4123	4010	3914	1543	407

Figure 4.1 Patients in the liraglutide arm had a statistically significant lower risk of the composite primary outcome than those in the placebo arm.

death from any cause was also lower in the liraglutide group (381 patients or 8.2%) versus placebo (447 patients or 9.6%) (HR [95% CI], 0.85 [0.74–0.97]; $p = .02$). The most common complaint among the liraglutide patients was gastrointestinal issues, and there was no increased risk of pancreatitis. Pre-specified microvascular outcome data from the LEADER trial indicate that liraglutide delays progression of renal events, in particular, new-onset persistent macroalbuminuria in patients with type 2 diabetes (Marso et al., 2016a). Evidence for cardiovascular protection with a, presently unlicensed, once weekly GLP-1 RA (semaglutide) has also recently been reported although this was a smaller, shorter duration study than LEADER and superiority for cardiovascular events was not a pre-specified endpoint (Marso et al., 2016b). The study adds to available data, however, which suggests both cardiovascular safety and benefit from this class of agents in patients with type 2 diabetes and cardiovascular disease. At the time of writing, similar studies with the other GLP-1 RAs are still awaited.

Exenatide should not be given to people with CKD stages 3–5 (GFR <60 mL/min) as it is eliminated by renal mechanisms. Data for the other GLP-1 RAs have been somewhat limited in patients with CKD, although both liraglutide and dulaglutide are now recommended as suitable in patients with mild to moderate renal impairment (down to eGFR 30 mL/min but not below).

Rates of adverse events differ between the individual agents, but the most common are gastrointestinal-related (nausea, vomiting and diarrhoea), which are transient and less common with the long-acting drugs. Injection site reactions may be more common with the long-acting agents, particularly exenatide once weekly which can cause transient small nodules at the injection site. Other long-acting agents show injection site reactions much less commonly and nodules are not a problem.

Pancreatitis has been reported in post-marketing surveillance for all marketed GLP-1 receptor agonists (as well as DPP-4 inhibitors). GLP-1 receptors are expressed in pancreatic islets and exocrine duct cells, and their stimulation can produce hyperplasia and chronic low-grade or acute inflammation in some experimental animal studies (Butler et al., 2013). In contrast, most epidemiological observational studies to date have reported relative risks of pancreatitis close to 1.0 among users of incretin-based (GLP-1 RA and DPP-4 inhibitors) versus other anti-diabetes drugs (Thomsen et al., 2015). The association of GLP-1 RAs with pancreatitis is difficult to assess because of the nearly threefold greater risk of pancreatitis in people with type 2 diabetes compared to those without type 2 diabetes (Noel et al., 2009). Obesity, smoking habits and alcohol consumption are additional risk factors. The issue of the relationship of incretins and acute pancreatitis therefore remains under debate. In patients with a history of pancreatitis (or people at high risk of pancreatitis, e.g. history of gall stones and alcoholism), glucose-lowering agents other than GLP-1 RAs should be used.

Although much research with the GLP-1 RAs focuses on increasing half-lives and extending injection intervals, there may be advantages of combining the short-acting agents with basal insulin preparations. Glycaemic control using insulin regimens is commonly attempted using basal insulin to target fasting plasma glucose, followed by the addition of bolus insulin to cover postprandial excursions. However, these types of intensive insulin regimens are associated with significant risks of hypoglycaemia and weight gain. The combination of basal insulin with a GLP-1 RA is a potential solution to this problem for some patients with type 2 diabetes: the basal insulin analogues targeting fasting and overall blood glucose, and the GLP-1 RA targeting post-prandial glucose at the same time as compensating for insulin-induced weight gain (Barnett, 2012). However, when added to insulin (or sulphonylureas), GLP-1 RAs are associated with an increased risk of hypoglycaemia so patients still need to be educated about this possibility. Additionally, whereas the basal insulin/GLP-1 RA combination literature has focussed more on the rapid acting GLP-1 RA agents, there is preliminary evidence that this combination also works well with the longer acting agents, including liraglutide and dulaglutide.

In the ADA/EASD 2015 guidelines, the GLP-1 RAs are recommended as a second-line therapy option in combination with metformin. They can also be used in combination with sulphonylureas, thiazolidinediones or basal insulin, providing a means of enhancing glucose control while offsetting weight gain. The latest NICE guidelines are more restrictive. A trial of combination therapy with metformin, a sulphonylurea and a GLP-1 RA may be offered to patients with high body mass index (BMI) who would otherwise require high doses of insulin. However, the opportunity to use GLP-1 RAs, despite strongly associated with weight loss, continues to be compromised by NICE thresholds for use (BMI $\geq$35 kg/m^2 or a BMI <35 kg/m^2 plus a comorbidity) and continuation criteria (HbA1c reduction $\geq$11 mmol/mol [1%] and weight loss $\geq$3% of initial body weight in 6 months). In clinical practice, some patients will show dramatic improvements in glycaemic control, but not lose 3% body weight, whereas others lose much weight, but do not quite reach the required 1% HbA1c reduction. Neither would meet the NICE criteria for continuing therapy, but both scenarios should be considered a clinical success.

An important point to add from the point of view of patient acceptability and treatment satisfaction is that all GLP-1 RAs are available for use with a pen injector and most are extremely easy to use.

Potential users of GLP-1 RAs

Overweight/obese, at risk for hypoglycaemia, willing to take injections, long-acting agents for people with irregular meal habits and lifestyles, unsuitable for or not wanting insulin, but failing to meet targets for glycaemic control with oral agents.

SGLT-2 inhibitors

The kidney plays an important role in glucose homeostasis by returning filtered glucose to the circulation and preventing its excretion in the urine. This is achieved in part by expression of SGLT-2 in the proximal renal tubule. SGLT-2 is responsible for reabsorption of approximately 90% of filtered glucose in the kidney. By limiting the actions of this transporter protein, the orally administered SGLT-2 inhibitors block the reabsorption of approximately 25%–30% of glucose in the kidneys (Figure 4.2). This promotes excretion of excess glucose in the urine, thereby lowering blood glucose. Loss of glucose in the urine means loss of calories so weight loss of around 2–3 kg is also predicted. Importantly, the

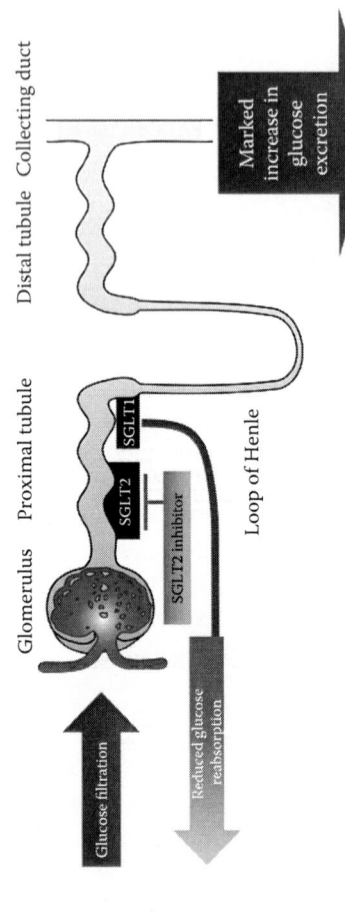

Figure 4.2 SGLT-2 inhibition lowers the inappropriately elevated renal threshold for glucose in type 2 diabetes. (Adapted from Bailey, C.J. et al., *Trends Pharmacol Sci*, 32, 63–71, 2011.)

mechanism of action of the SGLT-2 inhibitors is not dependent on functioning β cells or insulin, and they are therefore an option for those with advanced type 2 diabetes, particularly if glycaemic control is inadequate with existing oral anti-diabetes agents. Their insulin-independent mechanism of action also predicts a very low risk of hypoglycaemia (unless used in combination with a drug that promotes hypoglycaemia) and the possibility that they can be usefully combined with any other antidiabetes agent with a different mechanism of action. Clinical trials (see below) have tested all these predictions with positive results.

The SGLT-2 inhibitors are effective when used alone or with other agents, and three highly selective SGLT-2 inhibitors have been approved for use: dapagliflozin, canagliflozin and empagliflozin. They can be used throughout the natural history of type 2 diabetes, including in combination with insulin therapy, and all three are available as fixed-dose combinations with metformin; empagliflozin is also available as a fixed dose with linagliptin.

In a meta-analysis of clinical trials comparing SGLT-2 inhibitors with placebo in 45 studies ($n = 11,232$) and with active comparators in 13 studies ($n = 5175$), the mean HbA1c difference compared with placebo was −0.66% (95% CI, −0.73% to −0.58%) and the mean difference compared with active comparators was −0.06% (95% CI, −0.18% to 0.05%) (Vasilakou et al., 2013). They are also associated with a weight loss of approximately 2–3 kg, a low risk of hypoglycaemia and a decrease in blood pressure of approximately 4 mmHg systolic and 2 mmHg diastolic (Baker et al., 2014).

Adverse reactions include genital mycotic infections and urinary tract infections, particularly in women. Less common adverse effects include hypotension, dizziness, back pain, dysuria, polyuria and dyslipidaemia. The FDA has added warnings to the labels of the SGLT-2 inhibitors about the drugs' risk of causing urinary tract infections and diabetic ketoacidosis (DKA). There is no evidence as yet that SGLT-2 inhibitors are the cause of the DKA, but given the mechanism of action of these drugs, it is important that patients maintain a state of hydration. Case reports have established that many cases of DKA are associated with off-label use of SGLT-2 inhibitors in type 1 diabetes, and such usage should be actively discouraged, at least until further information is available. In addition, it is clear that a proportion of patients developing DKA have been wrongly diagnosed as having type 2 diabetes when in fact (on appropriate testing) they turn out to have slowly progressive type 1 diabetes of adults (Latent Autoimmune Diabetes of Adults [LADA]). Any patient who is not obese and who has rapidly progressive symptoms not responding well to oral therapy must be considered as possibly having LADA, which can be confirmed by appropriate pancreatic autoantibody tests.

As the efficacy of SGLT-2 inhibitors is dependent on renal function, their ability to lower blood glucose in patients with CKD is reduced. At present, only few studies have evaluated the effect of SGLT-2 inhibition in CKD. For this reason, their use is not recommended in subjects with severe renal impairment or end-stage renal disease. Of the available agents, dapagliflozin is not recommended to be used at eGFR below 60 mL/min. Canagliflozin and empagliflozin should not be initiated if eGFR is below 60 mL/min, but where patients are started above this level, they can be continued (at a lower dose) until eGFR falls below 45 mL/min. Dose adjustment may also be required in the elderly, and those on loop diuretics if there are concerns or symptoms of volume-related side effects (hypotension, dizziness, fainting).

Empagliflozin has recently been shown to reduce cardiovascular events and mortality over and above effects on glucose lowering in a long-term cardiovascular outcome trial. The EMPA-REG OUTCOME trial compared empagliflozin with placebo on cardiovascular morbidity and mortality in patients with type 2 diabetes and established cardiovascular disease receiving standard care, including statins, angiotensin converting enzyme inhibitors and aspirin. Over 7000 patients were randomized (1:1:1 to empagliflozin 10 mg or 25 mg or placebo once daily) and treated for a median of 2.6 years with a median observation time of 3.1 years (Zinman et al., 2015). The primary outcome of a composite of cardiovascular death, non-fatal MI or non-fatal stroke occurred in a significantly lower percentage of patients on empagliflozin (490 of 4687, 10.5%) than in the placebo group (282 of 2333, 12.1%, HR: 0.86, 95% CI: 0.74–0.99, $p < .001$ for non-inferiority and $p = .04$ for superiority). Empagliflozin showed a statistically significant

38% relative risk reduction in cardiovascular mortality and a 32% risk reduction in all-cause mortality as well as a significant 35% reduction in hospitalization for heart failure.

A secondary outcome of the EMPA-REG Outcome trial was a composite microvascular outcome that included the development or worsening of nephropathy. The endpoint occurred in 525/4124 empagliflozin-treated patients (12.7%) compared with 388/2061 placebo-treated patients (18.8%), a reduction of 39% (HR: 0.61, $p < .001$) (Wanner et al., 2016). Findings such as this may offer further opportunities for individualizing therapy for people with type 2 diabetes in relation to their underlying disease profile.

In the ADA/EASD 2015 guidelines, SGLT-2 inhibitors can be considered for dual therapy with metformin if blood glucose levels are not controlled on metformin monotherapy and also as triple therapy or in combination with insulin. NICE 2015 guidance states that treatment with combinations of drugs, including SGLT-2 inhibitors, may be appropriate for some people at first and second intensification and in combination with insulin.

The efficacy and safety package of SGLT-2 inhibitors looks extremely promising with significant reductions in glycaemia, weight loss, low risk of hypoglycaemia, blood pressure reductions, ability to combine with other anti-diabetes agents and most recently the exciting potential for cardiovascular protection in individuals with type 2 diabetes and established cardiovascular disease. The mechanism of cardiovascular protection is much debated, but given that the mortality curves separate almost immediately the assumption must be that this is likely to be a haemodynamic effect (perhaps by reducing risks of overt and incipient heart failure, both of which have a very high cardiovascular mortality) rather than any effects on glycaemia or weight loss.

Potential users of SGLT-2 inhibitors

Suitable for use at any stage of type 2 diabetes, overweight/ obese, problems with dietary adherence, at risk for hypoglycaemia, cardiovascular risk factors and specifically for those with established cardiovascular disease.

COMBINATION THERAPY WITH NEWER AGENTS

In addition to blood glucose control, the newer anti-diabetes agents have been developed to address many of the unmet needs in diabetes management such as weight gain, hypoglycaemia, complex dose regimens and lack of cardiovascular outcome data. From the patient's perspective, weight gain and hypoglycaemia are undesirable and unwanted side effects. Of the older therapies, sulphonylureas, pioglitazone and insulin are all associated with significant weight gain. As the majority of people with type 2 diabetes are overweight or obese, agents that offer a reduction in weight or weight loss combined with a low risk of hypoglycaemia would offer significant advantages as second-line therapy to metformin. Table 4.2 lists currently available anti-diabetes agents and indicates which classes can be used in combination.

Cardiovascular risk reduction also represents an important clinical goal in the light of the elevated risk of cardiovascular morbidity and mortality in the type 2 diabetes population. It is therefore important that anti-diabetes drugs have no negative effects on cardiovascular risk. With the newer treatment options available, therapy can now be tailored to those at high risk of cardiovascular events with the SGLT-2 inhibitor empagliflozin, even demonstrating significant improvements in cardiovascular outcomes. The benefits of the newer agents for type 2 diabetes have been further enhanced by the development of fixed-dose combinations, including DPP-4 inhibitors with metformin, SGLT-2 inhibitors with metformin and DPP-4 inhibitors with SGLT-2 inhibitors. In addition to additive effects on blood glucose lowering, combining agents with complementary mechanisms of action targets different pathophysiological pathways, reduces the risk of adverse events compared with higher dose monotherapy, and simplifies treatment regimens and improves adherence. These attributes add to the advantage of other benefits of the individual drugs such as improved β-cell sensitivity and/or cardiovascular benefits. The newer agents can also be used with insulin to bridge the gap in patients reluctant to initiate multiple daily injections of insulin. Such an approach takes advantage of the different mechanisms of action of the different treatments at the same time as counteracting insulin-associated weight gain.

Table 4.2 Classes of anti-diabetes agents and their use in combination

	Metformin	SU	Glinide	TZD	Alpha-glucosidase inhibitor	DPP-4 inhibitor	GLP-1 RA	SGLT-2 inhibitor
Metformin		✓	✓	✓	✓	✓	✓	✓
SU	✓		×	✓	×	✓	✓	✓ (lower SU dose)
Glinide	✓	×		×	×	×	×	×
TZD	✓	✓	×		×	✓	✓	✓
Alpha-glucosidase inhibitor	✓	×	×	×				
DPP-4 inhibitor	✓	✓	×	✓			×	✓
GLP-1 RA	✓	✓	×	✓		×		✓
SGLT-2 inhibitor	✓	✓ (lower SU dose)	×	✓		✓	✓	

SU, sulphonylureas; TZD, thiazolidinediones.

REFERENCES

Baker WL, Smyth LR, Riche DM, Bourret EM, Chamberlin KW, White WB. Effects of sodium-glucose co-transporter 2 inhibitors on blood pressure: A systematic review and meta-analysis. *J Am Soc Hypertens* 2014;8:262–275.

Bailey CJ. Renal glucose reabsorption inhibitors to treat diabetes. *Trends Pharmacol Sci* 2011;32:63–71.

Barnett AH. The role of GLP-1 mimetics and basal insulin analogues in type 2 diabetes mellitus: Guidance from studies of liraglutide. *Diabetes Obes Metab* 2012;14:304–314.

Butler AE, Campbell-Thompson M, Gurlo T, Dawson DW, Atkinson M, Butler PC. Marked expansion of exocrine and endocrine pancreas with incretin therapy in humans with increased exocrine pancreas dysplasia and the potential for glucagon-producing neuroendocrine tumors. *Diabetes* 2013;62:2595–2604.

Chilton RJ. Potential cardiovascular effects of the glucagon-like peptide-1 receptor agonists. *J Diabetes Metab* 2015;6:1.

Ekström N, Schiöler L, Svensson AM, Eeg-Olofsson K, Miao Jonasson J, Zethelius B, Cederholm J, Eliasson B, Gudbjörnsdottir S. Effectiveness and safety of metformin in 51,675 patients with type 2 diabetes and different levels of renal function: A cohort study from the Swedish National Diabetes Register. *BMJ Open* 2012;2(4). pii: e001076.

Ekström N, Svensson AM, Miftaraj M, Andersson Sundell K, Cederholm J, Zethelius B, Eliasson B, Gudbjörnsdottir S. Durability of oral hypoglycemic agents in drug naïve patients with type 2 diabetes: Report from the Swedish National Diabetes Register (NDR). *BMJ Open Diabetes Res Care* 2015;3:e000059.

Filion KB, Azoulay L, Platt RW et al.; CNODES Investigators. A multicenter observational study of incretin-based drugs and heart failure. *N Engl J Med* 2016;374:1145–1154.

Green JB, Bethel MA, Armstrong PW et al.; TECOS Study Group. Effect of sitagliptin on cardiovascular outcomes in type 2 diabetes. *N Engl J Med* 2015;373:232–242.

Inzucchi SE, Lipska KJ, Mayo H, Bailey CJ, McGuire DK. Metformin in patients with type 2 diabetes and kidney disease a systematic review. *JAMA* 2014;312:2668–2675.

Madsbad S. Review of head-to-head comparisons of glucagon-like peptide-1 receptor agonists. *Diabetes Obes Metab* 2016;18:317–332.

Marso SP, Daniels GH, Brown-Frandsen K et al.; on behalf of the LEADER Trial Investigators. Liraglutide and cardiovascular outcomes in type 2 diabetes. *N Engl J Med* 2016;375:311–322.

Marso SP, Bain SC, Consoli A et al.; SUSTAIN-6 Investigators. Semaglutide and cardiovascular outcomes in patients with type 2 diabetes. *N Engl J Med* 2016b. Epub ahead of print.

Meier JJ. GLP-1 receptor agonists for individualized treatment of type 2 diabetes mellitus. *Nature Rev Endocrinol* 2012;8:728–742.

Monami M, Iacomelli I, Marchionni N, Mannucci E. Dipeptidyl peptidase-4 inhibitors in type 2 diabetes: A meta-analysis of randomized clinical trials. *Nutr Metab Cardiovasc Dis* 2010;20:224–235.

National Institute for Health and Care Excellence. Type 2 diabetes in adults: Management. Clinical Guideline Update (NG28). Methods, evidence and recommendations, December 2015. Available from: https://www.nice.org.uk/guidance/ng28. Last accessed March 2016.

Noel RA, Braun DK, Patterson RE, Bloomgren GL. Increased risk of acute pancreatitis and biliary disease observed in patients with type 2 diabetes: A retrospective cohort study. *Diabetes Care* 2009;32:834–838.

Pfeffer MA, Claggett B, Diaz R et al.; ELIXA Investigators. Lixisenatide in patients with type 2 diabetes and acute coronary syndrome. *N Engl J Med* 2015;373:2247–2257.

Phung OJ, Scholle JM, Talwar M, Coleman CI. Effect of non-insulin antidiabetic drugs added to metformin therapy on glycemic control, weight gain, and hypoglycemia in type 2 diabetes. *JAMA* 2010;303:1410–1418.

Scirica BM, Bhatt DL, Braunwald E et al.; SAVOR-TIMI 53 Steering Committee and Investigators. Saxagliptin and cardiovascular outcomes in patients with type 2 diabetes mellitus. *N Engl J Med* 2013;369:1317–1326.

Tahrani AA, Barnett AH, Bailey CJ. Pharmacology and therapeutic implications of current drugs for type 2 diabetes mellitus. *Nat Rev Endocrinol* 2016;12:566–592.

Thomsen RW, Pedersen L, Møller N, Kahlert J, Beck-Nielsen H, Sørensen HT. Incretin-based therapy and risk of acute pancreatitis: A nationwide population-based case-control study. *Diabetes Care* 2015;38:1089–1098.

Vasilakou D, Karagiannis T, Athanasiadou E, Mainou M, Liakos A, Bekiari E, Sarigianni M, Matthews DR, Tsapas A. Sodium-glucose cotransporter 2 inhibitors for type 2 diabetes: A systematic review and meta-analysis. *Ann Intern Med* 2013;159:262–274.

Wanner C, Inzucchi SE, Lachin JM et al.; EMPA-REG OUTCOME Investigators. Empagliflozin and progression of kidney disease in type 2 diabetes. *N Engl J Med* 2016;375:323–334.

White WB, Cannon CP, Heller SR et al.; EXAMINE Investigators. Alogliptin after acute coronary syndrome in patients with type 2 diabetes. *N Engl J Med* 2013;369:1327–1335.

Zinman B, Wanner C, Lachin JM et al.; EMPA-REG OUTCOME Investigators. Empagliflozin, cardiovascular outcomes, and mortality in type 2 diabetes. *N Engl J Med* 2015;373:2117–2128.

5

New insulin developments

Insulin has traditionally been considered a treatment of last resort for individuals with type 2 diabetes, delayed until all other efforts by the patient and healthcare provider have failed. As β-cell function declines over time, the need for replacement insulin will increase in order to normalise blood glucose levels. β-cell decline can occur due to a number of factors, and the rate of β-cell decline and the degree of insulin resistance will be different for each individual. As a result, the right time to begin insulin will differ from person to person. In recognition of this, recent treatment guidelines recommend the use of insulin, in particular basal insulin, as part of a treatment regimen earlier in the disease process.

Insulin should not be seen as the last resort in optimising glycaemic control or as failure by the patient to control their diabetes, but rather as an option to optimise blood glucose control to prevent longer term complications. As many people are reluctant to commence multiple daily injections, insulin initiation often involves basal-only therapy in conjunction with existing oral anti-diabetes medications. Advantages of this approach include reduced risk of weight gain, reduced risk of hypoglycaemia, a simpler treatment regimen and better blood glucose control during insulin initiation and dose adjustments. Thereafter, insulin regimens that are more tailored to individual needs are likely to result in greater acceptance and patient adherence. To meet this need, a range of new insulins and insulin combinations have been developed that aim to prolong the duration of action of basal insulins; shorten the time to peak action of rapid-acting insulins; reduce peak variability, hypoglycaemia and weight gain; and provide greater flexibility in dosing time from day to day.

BASAL INSULINS

When initiating insulin therapy in a patient who is already on oral anti-diabetes medication, a basal (long- or intermediate-acting) insulin can be chosen to improve nocturnal and fasting blood glucose. Combining a glucagon-like peptide 1 receptor agonist (GLP-1 RA) with basal insulin is also an effective regimen for improving glycaemic control without increasing the risk of hypoglycaemia or weight gain (Vora et al., 2013). The basal insulin options of insulin neutral protamine hagedorn (NPH), glargine and detemir, have recently been joined by an insulin glargine biosimilar and the new ultra-long-acting basal insulins, insulin degludec and glargine U300 (Table 5.1).

Biosimilar insulins

Biosimilar insulins are the insulin equivalent of lower cost generic drugs, and several are in development for launch after the patents on analogue insulins expire. In contrast to drugs with relatively simple chemical structures, where generic copies can be produced by chemical synthesis, the complex structure of human insulin and its analogues means that similar versions can only be manufactured by a biotechnological approach using genetically modified bacteria and yeast. The biological conditions in which the insulin is manufactured, such as the incubation conditions in different laboratories using slightly different strains of bacteria and yeast, will lead to the production of similar, but not identical insulins (Heinemann, 2012).

The first such insulin to become available is biosimilar insulin glargine. This has demonstrated similar pharmacodynamics and pharmacokinetics and a similar safety and efficacy profile to insulin glargine (Rosenstock et al., 2015b). The National Institute for

Table 5.1 Long-acting insulin analogues

Preparation	Dosage form	Pharmacokinetics		
		Onset of action (h)	Duration of action (h)	Peak effect (h)
Humulin® N (NPH)	Vial (100 U/mL) 10 mL vial Pen—KwikPen® (100 U/mL) 3 mL pen	2–4	up to 20	4–10
Novolin® N (NPH)	Vial (100 U/mL) 10 mL vial	2–4	up to 20	4–10
Lantus® (insulin glargine)	Vial (100 U/mL) 10 ml vial Pen – SoloStar® (100 U/mL) 3 ml pen	1–3	24+	No peak
Toujeo® (insulin glargine)	Pen—SoloStar® (300 U/mL) 1.5 mL pen	6	24+	No peak
Abasaglar® (biosimilar insulin glargine)	Pen—KwikPen® (100 U/mL) 3 mL pen	1–3	24+	No peak
Levemir® (insulin detemir)	Vial (100 U/mL) 10 mL vial Pen—FlexPen® (100 U/mL) 3 mL pen Pen—FlexTouch® (100 U/mL) 3 mL pen	1–3	6–24 (depends on dose)	Varies
Tresiba® (insulin degludec)	Pen—FlexTouch® U-100 = 100 U/mL U-200 = 200 U/mL 3 mL pens	1–3	24+	No peak

Health and Care Excellence (NICE) position statement on biosimilars states that NICE guidance on a product also applies to relevant licensed biosimilar products, which subsequently appear on the market. However, in the first instance, it may be appropriate to limit biosimilar insulin treatment to new patients or patients assessed as needing a medication change until clinical experience of the treatment and its delivery device has been gained. Insulin glargine and biosimilar insulin glargine use slightly different delivery devices.

Insulin degludec

The active form of insulin is the monomer, but insulin is produced and stored in the body as a hexamer, an inactive form with long-term stability. Manipulation of the hexamer-to-monomer conversion is central to the development of new insulin analogues. Insulin degludec is an ultra-long-acting insulin with a half-life of more than 24 h and a duration of action of more than 42 h. It forms stable dihexamers in solution in the presence of phenol and zinc. After injection, the phenol dissipates and the dihexamers begin to associate with each other to form long multi-hexamer chains. The slow diffusion of zinc from the end of these multi-hexamers causes a gradual, continuous and extended release of insulin monomers from the injection site without any significant peaks that would cause unpredictable blood sugars (Jonassen et al., 2012). Compared with insulin glargine and detemir, degludec has a flatter pharmacokinetic and pharmacodynamic profile, decreasing the number of confirmed hypoglycaemia episodes, particularly nocturnal hypoglycaemia (Ratner et al., 2013).

Insulin degludec has been extensively studied in the BEGIN® programme, which covered the spectrum of people with diabetes who require insulin treatment (insulin-naive type 2 diabetes, insulin-treated type 2 and type 1 diabetes including basal–bolus therapy, basal plus oral therapy and basal vs. oral therapy, and also the flexible dosing options). Although insulin degludec provides similar blood glucose control to NPH insulin, glargine and detemir, it is able to address some of the concerns around initiation of insulin therapy. A pre-planned meta-analysis of phase III trials has shown that subjects with type 2 diabetes who were treated with insulin degludec experienced significantly lower rates of overall confirmed (lower by 17%) and nocturnal confirmed hypoglycaemic episodes (lower by 32%) compared with insulin glargine ($p < .05$) (Ratner et al., 2013). Results were similar in insulin-experienced and insulin-naive patients.

An additional advantage of insulin degludec is that it may be given at any time of day (although preferably at the same time every day), and administration time can vary from day to day without compromising efficacy or safety (a minimum of 8 h between injections should always be ensured). The ability to exercise greater flexibility in dosing schedules may help to lessen the effects of irregular insulin dosing and appeal to people with hectic lifestyles who would find it difficult to adhere to a strict dosing schedule, or to those reluctant to intensify to insulin treatment because of perceptions about the restrictiveness of the regimen.

Insulin degludec can be used both as a basal regime and as part of a basal–bolus regime. It is also available as a fixed-ratio combination with the GLP-1 RA liraglutide. This is administered as once-daily subcutaneous injections, which for some people may be preferable to giving basal insulin and GLP-1 RAs separately. The combination product was associated with a mean weight loss of 2.2–2.5 kg from baseline compared with insulin degludec alone, but 2.4 kg less weight loss compared with liraglutide alone (Gough et al., 2014). The dose is administered in dose steps, with one 'step' containing 1 unit of insulin degludec and 0.036 mg liraglutide. As it is a fixed-ratio combination product, it is not possible to titrate the dose of basal insulin and liraglutide separately. The advantage of a set dose ratio is that it reduces the risk of errors in dialling up an incorrect dose or the risk of confusing injector pens.

Glargine U300

The most recent clinical approach for ultra-long insulin is glargine 300 U/mL (U300). This formulation uses the same mechanisms to extend absorption as regular insulin glargine 100 U/mL, but once injected, the new high-strength formulation forms a compact subcutaneous depot with a smaller surface area than regular glargine resulting in a more gradual and prolonged release and flatter pharmacokinetic and pharmacodynamic profile. Exposure to glargine U300 is more evenly distributed and blood glucose control is maintained for up to 36 h.

The efficacy and safety of glargine U300 compared with regular glargine has been studied in the EDITION clinical trial programme, which consisted of three randomised, open-label trials in people with type 2 diabetes and one trial in people with type 1 diabetes. Trials were 6 months in duration with 6-month extensions. Of the type 2 diabetes trials, two were add-on to oral agents and the other was add-on to prandial insulin ± metformin. In the 6-month EDITION trials, glargine U300 consistently demonstrated blood glucose control comparable to regular glargine. However, the 12-month data for EDITION 1 (prandial insulin ± metformin) showed a significantly greater reduction in haemoglobin A1c (HbA1c) with glargine U300 than regular glargine (0.86% vs. 0.69%). In the type 2 diabetes EDITION trials, those receiving glargine U300 required 11%–15% more basal insulin than those receiving regular glargine.

It has been speculated that the smoother pharmacokinetic and pharmacodynamic profile of glargine U300 may result in a lower risk of hypoglycaemia, and in general, there was a tendency towards less hypoglycaemia with glargine U300 (Ritzel et al., 2015). There was also evidence for less weight gain with glargine U300 compared with regular insulin, despite a higher insulin dose. Mean weight changes in a pooled analysis of the three type 2 diabetes trials were 0.51 and 0.79 kg for glargine U300 and regular glargine, respectively (Ritzel et al., 2015).

Glargine U300 and regular insulin glargine are not bioequivalent and not interchangeable without dose adjustment. When switching to or from glargine U300, close monitoring is recommended during the transition and the initial weeks to reduce the risk of hypoglycaemia. Glargine U300 is available in a pen form only calibrated to dispense the expected dose. This is to eliminate the possibility of accidentally using a syringe calibrated for regular glargine 100 U/mL and injecting 3 times as much glargine U300 as required with serious hypoglycaemic consequences. Glargine

U300 may be a useful option in individuals who currently inject basal insulin twice daily, as it can be given once daily in a smaller volume, with the potential for less night-time hypoglycaemia and less weight gain. It may also be a good option to add on to oral anti-diabetes therapy in people who would benefit from the addition of background insulin. The safety profile of glargine U300 is similar to regular glargine, and the EDITION trials found no evidence of increased injection site problems.

RAPID-ACTING INSULIN ANALOGUES

Ultra-rapid-acting insulin analogues

The rapid-acting insulin analogues insulin aspart, lispro and glulisine were developed to more closely approach the physiological insulin response, compared with regular human insulin, and represented a step forward in post-prandial glucose control. However, an injection–meal interval of around 30 min is still required to achieve optimum post-prandial glucose control. Formulations with an even more rapid onset of action and a shorter duration of action that would better match the rapid rise in blood glucose that follows meals would give people more flexibility in their daily schedules, and potentially less hypoglycaemia.

A rapid increase in circulating insulin levels can be achieved by a number of different methods, including modification of the primary structure of the insulin molecule, addition of excipients that result in more rapid dissociation of insulin hexamere into active monomers, addition of enzymes such as hyaluronidase to enable more rapid spreading of the insulin molecules in subcutaneous tissue, and increasing the insulin absorption rate by improving local blood flow in the injection zone.

A number of ultra-rapid-acting insulins are in development, but the most advanced is currently faster acting insulin aspart (FIAsp), which contains the excipients nicotinamide and L-arginine to speed up monomer formation (Heise et al., 2015). Onset of appearance in the bloodstream is twice as fast and exposure within the first 30 min is twofold higher compared with regular aspart (Heise et al., 2015). Regulatory approval in both Europe and the United

States was filed in December 2015 based on the results from the ONSET clinical trial programme, which involved approximately 2100 adults with type 1 and type 2 diabetes. In these trials, people treated with FIAsp achieved improvements in post-prandial control versus regular insulin aspart with similar HbA1c reductions. Across the ONSET trials, FIAsp was safe and well tolerated, with the most common adverse event being hypoglycaemia, similar to the levels observed with regular insulin aspart.

Inhaled insulin

An alternative method of rapidly increasing circulating insulin levels is to administer insulin via the lungs. Technosphere-inhaled insulin (Afrezza®) delivers insulin to the lungs in microparticles using a small and convenient inhaler. The insulin powder is supplied in a single-use cartridge and is designed to be inhaled at the start of a meal or within 20 min and achieves peak insulin levels in 12–15 min. In people with type 2 diabetes, the efficacy and safety of the inhaled insulin in combination with oral anti-diabetes drugs has been compared with placebo inhalation in a 24-week study. Inhaled insulin reduced HbA1c by −0.8% (−9.0 mmol/mol) from a baseline of 8.3% (66.8 mmol/mol) compared with placebo inhalation −0.4% (−4.6 mmol/mol) ($p < .0001$) (Rosenstock et al., 2015a). Mild, transient dry cough was the most common adverse event.

The concept of delivering insulin directly to the lungs broadens the options available for delivering mealtime insulin and may be beneficial for those with needle phobias. It has been approved for use by the U.S. Food and Drug Administration, but is not yet licensed in the United Kingdom or Europe. Use of inhaled insulin is not recommended in those who smoke, and it is contraindicated in patients with chronic obstructive pulmonary disease or asthma because of the increased risk of acute bronchospasm.

CONCLUSIONS

The management of type 2 diabetes requires an appreciation of its variable and progressive nature, the patient and disease factors that drive clinical decision making and the specific role of each drug in individualized, patient-centred care. A range of new therapies both oral and injectable are now available to help people reach their blood glucose targets with a low risk of hypoglycaemia and reduced weight gain. Several promising new insulin products and technologies have also been developed to address some of the current barriers to insulin initiation and intensification that currently limit the effectiveness of diabetes care.

REFERENCES

Gough SC, Bode B, Woo V et al.; NN9068-3697 (DUAL-I) Trial Investigators. Efficacy and safety of a fixed-ratio combination of insulin degludec and liraglutide (IDegLira) compared with its components given alone: Results of a phase 3, open-label, randomised, 26-week, treat-to-target trial in insulin-naive patients with type 2 diabetes. *Lancet Diabetes Endocrinol* 2014;2:885–893.

Heinemann L. Biosimilar insulins. *Expert Opin Biol Ther* 2012;12:1009–1016.

Heise T, Hövelmann U, Brøndsted L, Adrian CL, Nosek L, Haahr H. Faster-acting insulin aspart: Earlier onset of appearance and greater early pharmacokinetic and pharmacodynamic effects than insulin aspart. *Diabetes Obes Metab* 2015;17:682–688.

Jonassen I, Havelund S, Hoeg-Jensen T, Steensgaard DB, Wahlund PO, Ribel U. Design of the novel protraction mechanism of insulin degludec, ultra-long-acting basal insulin. *Pharm Res* 2012;29:2104–2114.

Ratner RE, Gough SC, Mathieu C, Del Prato S, Bode B, Mersebach H, Endahl L, Zinman B. Hypoglycaemia risk with insulin degludec compared with insulin glargine in type 2 and type 1 diabetes: A pre-planned meta-analysis of phase 3 trials. *Diabetes Obes Metab* 2013;15:175–184.

Ritzel, R, Roussel R, Bolli GB et al. Patient-level meta-analysis, of EDITION 1, 2, 3: Glycemic control and hypoglycemia with new insulin glargine 300 U/mL versus glargine 100 U/mL in people with type 2 diabetes. *Diabetes Obes Metab* 2015;17:859–867.

Rosenstock J, Franco D, Korpachev V, Shumel B, Ma Y, Baughman R, Amin N, McGill JB; Affinity 2 Study Group. Inhaled Technosphere Insulin versus Inhaled Technosphere Placebo in insulin-naïve subjects with type 2 diabetes inadequately controlled on oral antidiabetes agents. *Diabetes Care* 2015a;38:2274–2281.

Rosenstock J, Hollander P, Bhargava A et al.; Similar efficacy and safety of LY2963016 insulin glargine and insulin glargine (Lantus®) in patients with type 2 diabetes who were insulin-naïve or previously treated with insulin glargine: A randomized, double-blind controlled trial (the ELEMENT 2 study). *Diabetes Obes Metab* 2015b;17:734–741.

Vora J, Bain SC, Damci T et al.; Incretin-based therapy in combination with basal insulin: A promising tactic for the treatment of type 2 diabetes. *Diabetes Metab* 2013;39:6–15.

6

Personalised management

Optimal management of individuals with type 2 diabetes involves complex decision-making to achieve and maintain control of blood glucose as well as other risk factors. The blueprint for care is generally considered the clinical practice guideline, which was developed to reduce inappropriate variations in practice and to promote the delivery of high-quality, evidence-based health care. The highest quality of evidence is generally considered to come from the randomised, controlled clinical trial. However, these are performed with the primary goal of understanding the efficacy of a therapy in a selected group of patients, which may perform differently in varying clinical settings and in broader patient populations than those studied in traditional randomised, controlled trials. The practice of evidence-based medicine should therefore integrate clinical information obtained from a patient with the best evidence available from clinical research and experience. The result is personalised management, a flexible, individual approach that considers important variables involved in a person's diabetes care. Strategies tailored to the particular characteristics of individual patients have a number of advantages (Table 6.1) and promise to maximally improve the health of the population by optimising outcomes for each individual. This approach is highlighted in both the updated National Institute

Table 6.1 Advantages of personalised care

- Shift the emphasis in medicine from reaction to prevention.
- Direct the selection of optimal therapy and reduce trial-and-error prescribing.
- Help avoid adverse drug reactions.
- Reduce the likelihood of clinical inertia by agreeing a realistic management plan.
- Increase patient adherence to treatment.
- Improve the quality of life.
- Help control the overall cost of health care.

for Health and Care Excellence (NICE) guidance (NICE, 2015) and the 2015 joint position statement from the American Diabetes Association (ADA) and the European Association for the Study of Diabetes (EASD) (Inzucchi et al., 2015).

FACTORS TO CONSIDER IN PERSONALISED DIABETES MANAGEMENT

When evaluating patients with type 2 diabetes and their individual characteristics and needs, there is no shortage of things to consider. What are the patient's age, weight and height? How long has he or she been living with the disease? What other medications have been tried and at what doses? How is the patient's kidney, liver and gastrointestinal function? What is their current haemoglobin A1c (HbA1c) and fasting glucose level? Does the patient have a history of good adherence to treatment? What about his or her motivation, education level, cultural and social history, literacy level, allergies and tolerance to medications?

After evaluating the patient, the question then becomes which one or combination of more than 13 classes of drugs is most appropriate? Do dosing changes need to be made based on the patient's kidney or liver function? Are there potential drug interactions with medications the patient is already taking? Does the patient know how to take, where to store and how to evaluate the effectiveness of the medications? Does he or she have the faculties and support to appropriately manage the selected regimen?

LIFESTYLE MANAGEMENT

In current clinical practice guidelines (including the recent NICE recommendations [NICE, 2015]), lifestyle advice ideally given as part of a structured education programme is recommended from diagnosis with regular reinforcement and review at least annually. However, a change in lifestyle warrants a change in behaviour, which is usually more difficult to implement than prescribing a therapy (it is easy to take a pill, but harder to change lifestyle for good) and is therefore often perceived as a less-effective method of managing diabetes. Nevertheless, the role of lifestyle modification should not be underestimated. The Health Care Professional should agree with the patient what lifestyle changes are realistic, are feasible and can be enacted. This should be the mainstay of a personalised lifestyle plan and is an integral part of diabetes management.

Pre-diabetes

Lifestyle intervention plays an important role in diabetes prevention, especially in high-risk groups such as those with impaired fasting glucose and/or impaired glucose tolerance in whom blood glucose levels fall between normal and those defining type 2 diabetes (pre-diabetes). Both the Finnish Prevention Study (Tuomilehto et al., 2001) and the Diabetes Prevention Program (DPP, 2003) demonstrated conclusively that intensive lifestyle interventions decreased the overall risk of diabetes by 58% in persons defined as having impaired glucose intolerance. In the Finnish Prevention Study, the rates of diabetes risk reduction were highest in people who achieved the greatest adherence to the following:

- Weight reduction >5%
- Fat intake <30% of total energy intake
- Saturated fat intake <10% of total energy intake
- Dietary fibre intake ≥15 g/1000 kcal
- At least moderate intensity exercise for >4 h/week

The beneficial effects were maintained long term, with the intervention group demonstrating a 43% reduction in risk of diabetes over an average of 7 years of follow-up (Lindström et al., 2006). In the intervention group, sustained lifestyle changes remained even after individual lifestyle counselling had ended.

Diagnosed type 2 diabetes

Early in the course of the disease and in individuals in whom insulin resistance is the major pathophysiological abnormality, either energy restriction or weight loss will improve blood glucose levels. Weight loss may be less effective in terms of blood glucose control in individuals with marked β-cell dysfunction, but lifestyle interventions should still be maintained to reduce cardiovascular disease risk factors and prevent weight gain. Visceral adiposity, in particular, and its accompanying inflammatory processes contribute significantly to increased insulin resistance and vascular complication progression (Neeland et al., 2012).

With a structured lifestyle intervention program, including energy restriction, regular physical activity and frequent contact with healthcare care professionals, the majority of individuals can expect to lose 5%–10% of their starting weight. The most successful nutritional strategy for prevention and treatment of type 2 diabetes is one that is personalised and that takes into consideration culture, food availability and personal preferences, but follows recommendations that encourage a variety of foods from the five main food groups each day: carbohydrates, protein, milk and dairy products, fruit and vegetables, fats and sugars. NICE recommends personalising recommendations for carbohydrate and alcohol intake, and meal patterns (NICE, 2015). In this respect, the best diets are those which work best for the individual – there is no 'one-size-fits-all approach'.

The goal is for adequate amounts of nutrients and calories to maintain ideal weight, help stabilise blood glucose levels and assist in the maintenance of an optimal lipid profile. Extreme dietary restriction and avoidance of certain food groups might achieve short-term weight loss, but do not represent a sustainable balanced diet plan. It is more likely that weight loss is associated with adherence to diet rather than a specific type of diet (Dansinger et al., 2005). If weight loss reaches a plateau, physicians should continue to encourage the same lifestyle strategies that led to weight loss to prevent the weight regain.

Physical activity acts independently and synergistically with attempts to control weight regain achieved through nutritional interventions and may improve glycaemic control (and particularly insulin resistance) without reducing body weight. Exercise is critical in reducing cardiovascular and mortality outcomes among patients with type 2 diabetes (Wei et al., 2000); low physical activity is associated with increased arterial stiffness in patients recently diagnosed with type 2 diabetes as well as healthy controls (Funck et al., 2015). Even brief interventions to increase the dialogue between patients and healthcare providers about behavioural goals have been shown to lead to increased physical activity and weight loss (Christian et al., 2008).

There is currently a lack of knowledge concerning the optimal lifestyle intervention programmes in type 2 diabetes to ensure both compliance and long-term health outcomes. This is being addressed by the ongoing U-TURN study, which is assessing the effects of an intensive lifestyle intervention on glycaemic control in patients with type 2 diabetes, and whether such interventions can decrease the need for anti-diabetes medications (Ried-Larsen et al., 2015).

Pharmacotherapy

In 2015, a number of institutions and societies published updated guidelines for the management of type 2 diabetes, including NICE and ADA/EASD (Inzucchi et al., 2015; NICE, 2015). Both NICE and ADA/EASD stress the importance of personalised management, but with some differences between them. Initial HbA1c targets in the NICE guidelines are 48 mmol/mol (6.5%) for those managed with lifestyle interventions alone or lifestyle combined with a drug not associated with hypoglycaemia; for those on a drug associated with hypoglycaemia, the target is 53 mmol/mol (7.0%). ADA/EASD do not put a specific HbA1c number in their position statement, but instead highlight patients in whom goals should be more or less stringent (Figure 6.1). The strategy remains step-up, with intensification

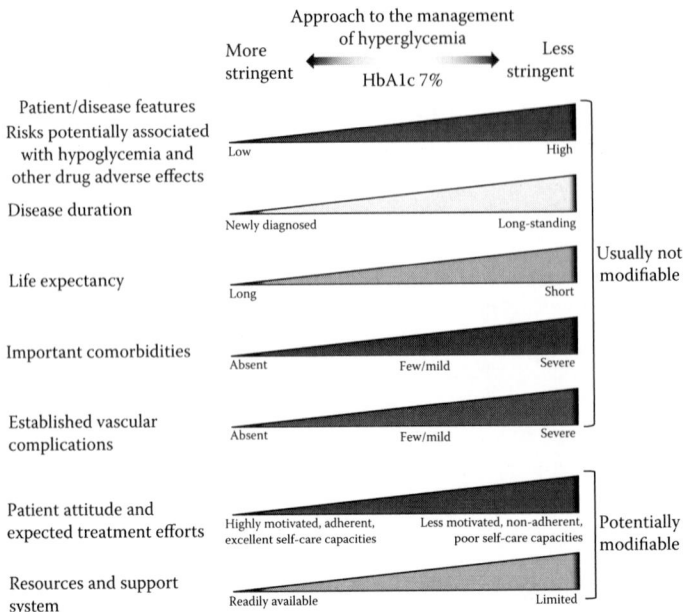

Figure 6.1 ADA/EASD depiction of patient and disease factors that may be used by the practitioner to determine optimal HbA1c targets in people with type 2 diabetes. Greater concerns about a particular domain are represented by increasing height of the ramp. Thus, characteristics/predicaments towards the left justify more stringent efforts to lower HbA1c, whereas those towards the right are compatible with less stringent efforts. (Reproduced from Inzucchi, S.E. et al., *Diabetes Care*, 38, 140–149, 2015. With permission.)

of drug or insulin dose. With NICE, this occurs when HbA1c levels are not adequately controlled by a single drug and rise to 58 mmol/L (7.5%) or higher. Unfortunately, this has echos of the old 'waiting-for-failure approach' and is totally inappropriate for many patients, particularly younger patients and in those more recently diagnosed. ADA/EASD advises treatment intensification if HbA1c targets are not achieved after approximately 3 months, whatever the initial target HbA1c, which seems a much more sensible approach.

As with past guidelines, there is an assumption that in each patient with type 2 diabetes, metformin is used initially (Figures 6.2 and 6.3a) (unless not tolerated or contraindicated [Figure 6.3b]). Second-line treatments are no longer prioritised (Figures 6.2 and 6.3a). ADA/EASD propose one of the six second-line treatment options (sulphonylurea, pioglitazone, dipeptidyl peptidase-4 (DPP-4) inhibitor, sodium–glucose cotransporter 2 [SGLT-2] inhibitor, GLP-1 receptor agonist [GLP-1 RA] or basal insulin) in combination with metformin (Figure 6.2). The NICE options in combination with metformin are a DPP-4 inhibitor, pioglitazone, sulphonylurea or an SGLT-2 inhibitor (Figure 6.3a).

Both guidelines highlight the need to personalise treatment targets as well as treatment strategies, with an emphasis on patient-centred care and shared decision-making. However, this is no easy task in a complex disease such as diabetes where personalised care means implementing a treatment strategy that is in line with the patient's preferences, specific risks and unique underlying disease pathophysiology and drug metabolism profile.

HbA1c targets should be decided with the patient after considering a number of factors, including age, current level of blood glucose control, duration of diabetes, comorbid conditions, risk of hypoglycaemia, patient motivation and ability to benefit from long-term interventions because of reduced life expectancy. Selection of the drug or drug combinations to help achieve this individual target is influenced by a number of factors as illustrated in Table 6.2.

Safety and efficacy should be given higher priorities than initial acquisition cost, as cost of medications forms only a small part of the total cost of diabetes care. In the United Kingdom, for example, therapies to treat diabetes are estimated to represent less than 8% of the total costs of the condition, with long-term complications accounting for over 80% (Table 6.3) (Kanavos et al., 2012).

The large number of available anti-diabetes therapies provides opportunities to tailor the regimen to patients' specific needs and preferences, which should be reassessed at each review. The guideline algorithms are the starting point for treatment.

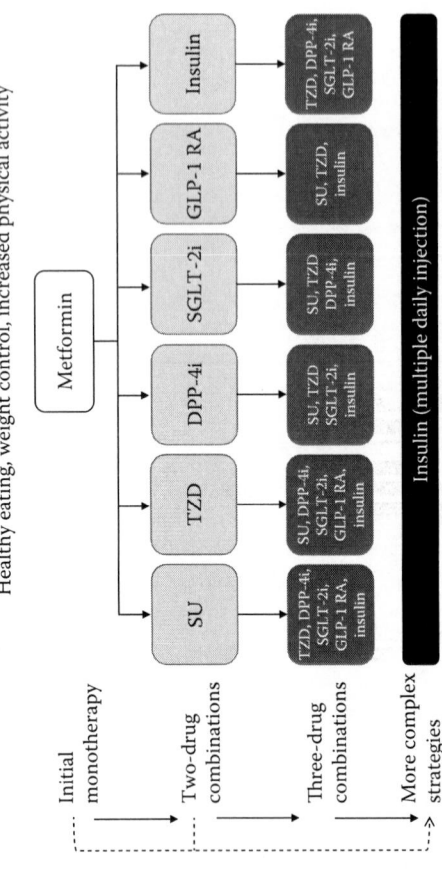

Figure 6.2 ADA/EASD 2015 algorithm for managing hyperglycaemia. SU, sulphonylurea; TZD, thiazolidinedione; DPP-4i, dipeptidyl peptidase 4 inhibitor; SGLT-2i; sodium–glucose cotransporter 2 inhibitor; GLP-1 RA, glucagon like peptide 1 receptor agonist. (Reproduced with permission from Inzucchi, S.E. et al., *Diabetes Care*, 38, 140–149, 2015. With permission.)

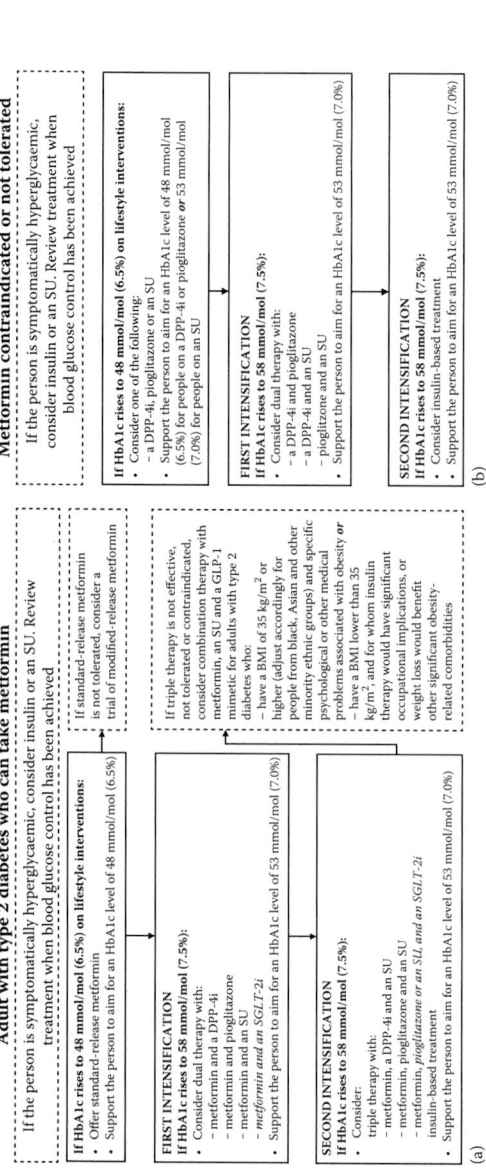

Figure 6.3 NICE update 2015 algorithm for blood glucose-lowering therapy in (a) adults with type 2 diabetes who can take metformin and (b) adults with type 2 diabetes in whom metformin is contraindicated or not tolerated. SU, sulphonylurea; DPP-4i, dipeptidyl peptidase 4 inhibitor; SGLT-2i, sodium–glucose cotransporter 2 inhibitor; GLP-1 RA, glucagon like peptide 1 receptor agonist. (National Institute for Health and Care Excellence, Type 2 diabetes in adults: Management. Clinical Guideline Update (NG28). Methods, evidence and recommendations. Available from: https://www.nice.org.uk/guidance/ng28, 2015.)

Table 6.2 Factors influencing choice of anti-diabetes therapy

Severity of hyperglycaemia

Stage of disease

Risk of inducing hypoglycaemia

Risk of weight gain

Ease of use

Cardiovascular risk profile

Safety impact on kidney, heart or liver disease

Risks from polypharmacy

Occupation and patient preferences

Table 6.3 Cost (£ billion) of diabetes treatment in the United Kingdom in 2012

Area of expenditure	Type 1 diabetes	Type 2 diabetes	Total cost	Percentage of costs
Diabetes drugs	£0.344	£0.712	£1.056	7.8
Non-diabetes drugs	£0.281	£1.810	£2.091	15.2
Inpatient	£1.007	£8.038	£9.045	65.8
Outpatient (excluding drugs)	£0.170	£1.158	£1.328	9.7
Other (including social service)	–	–	£0.230	1.7
Total	£1.802	£11.718	£13.750	100

Source: Kanavos, P. et al., *Diabetes expenditure, burden of disease and management in 5 EU countries*, London School of Economics, 2012; Diabetes UK.

To personalise care, management decisions for each individual then need to effectively address a series of questions:

- Based on the observed phenotype, how does the guideline recommendation apply to this individual?
- Are recommended therapies concordant with other conditions?
- If recommended treatment does not apply, how does it need to be modified?
- Do the predicted treatment benefits outweigh any risks?

The following case studies illustrate how the above questions can be applied to the NICE and ADA/EASD guidelines to determine optimal care for an individual.

CASE STUDY 6.1: A 55-YEAR-OLD MALE BUS DRIVER DIAGNOSED WITH TYPE 2 DIABETES 3 YEARS AGO

- Strong family history of coronary heart disease (CHD). Body mass index (BMI) 28 kg/m^2, normal renal function.
- Despite more lifestyle advice, HbA1c has crept up to 7.5% (58 mmol/mol).
- Drugs: statin and anti-hypertensives, plus metformin 1000 mg bd.

Based on the observed phenotype, how does the guideline recommendation apply to this individual?

Individual is already on a good daily dose of metformin (little dose response beyond 1000 mg bd but significant increase in gastrointestinal side effects at doses higher than this) and has had a steadily increasing HbA1c making him appropriate for treatment intensification in both guidelines. Particularly relevant in this respect is his relatively young age and short duration of disease.

Are recommended therapies concordant with other conditions?

The individual's occupation means that sulphonylureas are not an appropriate option because of the physician's concerns about the risk of hypoglycaemia (and indeed weight gain). Pioglitazone is not a good option as it could cause further weight gain plus risks of fluid retention and possibly even heart failure should he have incipient cardiovascular disease (CVD). DPP-4 inhibitors are possible options with the advantage of very low risk of hypoglycaemia in combination with metformin and weight neutrality. SGLT-2 inhibitors are also possible options with the added potential of weight loss, low risk of hypoglycaemia and blood pressure reduction. GLP-1 RAs are not a recommended dual therapy option in the NICE guideline, but could be used if following the ADA/EASD guideline. They are injectable, but have the advantage again of weight loss and low risk of hypoglycaemia.

Do the predicted treatment benefits outweigh any risks?

In the current scenario, the physician's preferred choice would be an SGLT-2 inhibitor as it has a very low risk of hypoglycaemia, would help with weight loss and has good efficacy. A DPP-4 inhibitor would be a reasonable alternative as it is very well tolerated, weight neutral and has low risk of hypoglycaemia.

CASE STUDY 6.2: AN 83-YEAR-OLD WOMAN WITH TYPE 2 DIABETES DIAGNOSED 10 YEARS AGO

- BMI 26 kg/m², estimated glomerular filtration rate (eGFR) 35 mL/min. Lives alone, angina, non-smoker.
- HbA1c 7.8% (62 mmol/mol), thirsty, nocturic, tired.
- Drugs: anti-anginals, simvastatin, metformin 500 mg bd.

Based on the observed phenotype, how does the guideline recommendation apply to this individual?

Patient is elderly with a number of comorbid conditions, and less stringent HbA1c target could be applied, except for the fact that she has symptoms.

Are recommended therapies concordant with other conditions?

As avoidance of hypoglycaemia is paramount in this elderly patient, a good case can be made for using a DPP-4 inhibitor, which has utility in a broad spectrum of patients.

Do the predicted treatment benefits outweigh any risks?

Linagliptin would be the physician's treatment of choice because it does not require dose adjustment (regardless of the extent of renal impairment) and also has established safety data in the elderly. Another DPP-4 inhibitor could be used provided dose adjustment is made to allow for her renal impairment.

CASE STUDY 6.3: A 46-YEAR-OLD MAN WITH TYPE 2 DIABETES DIAGNOSED 3 YEARS AGO

- BMI 27 kg/m^2, hypertension, background retinopathy and microalbuminuria. Now very symptomatic.
- HbA1c progressive deterioration and now 9.3% (78 mmol/mol).
- Drugs: metformin 1000 mg bd, simvastatin 40 mg once daily, ramipril 10 mg once daily, indapamide 2.5 mg once daily.

Based on the observed phenotype, how does the guideline recommendation apply to this individual?

Because this overweight individual with type 2 diabetes has marked symptoms of poor control, including HbA1c 9.3% and rapidly progressive long-term complications, insulin therapy is required. Also note here the possibility of type 1 diabetes, that is, Latent Autoimmune Diabetes of Adults, which can be confirmed by the presence of islet-related antibodies.

CASE STUDY 6.4: A 68-YEAR-OLD WOMAN WITH TYPE 2 DIABETES DIAGNOSED 8 YEARS AGO

- BMI 33 kg/m^2, hypertension, dyslipidaemia, hypothyroidism.
- HbA1c 8.4% (68 mmol/mol), eGFR 46 mL/min.
- Drugs: cardioprotective agents, thyroxine 125 µg/day, metformin 1000 mg bd, gliclazide 80 mg bd.

Based on the observed phenotype, how does the guideline recommendation apply to this individual?

Individual is already on dual therapy with good daily dose of metformin and has an HbA1c of 8.4% making her appropriate for treatment intensification.

Are recommended therapies concordant with other conditions?

The sulphonylurea dose could be increased, but there is little dose response of this class of agents beyond half the recommended maximum dose (which this lady is already taking), but may lead to a higher risk of hypoglycaemia (particularly in a renal-impaired patient who is therefore already at high risk of hypoglycaemic events) and weight gain.

Adding pioglitazone is a triple therapy option recommended by NICE and may help control HbA1c, but may exacerbate weight problems and should be used with great caution in patients with a history of CVD because of concerns regarding fluid retention and heart failure. There is also an increased risk of bone fractures, particularly in women.

Insulin is an option, but concerns around hypoglycaemia and weight gain would mitigate against its use. SGLT-2 inhibitor therapy is contraindicated in individuals with an eGFR below 60 mL/min.

If recommended treatment does not apply, how does it need to be modified?

Adding a DPP-4 inhibitor is a triple therapy option recommended by NICE, but would be associated with a higher risk of hypogly-caemia in combination with the sulphonylurea (for this reason, it would be wise to reduce the sulphonylurea dose). DPP-4 inhibi-tors are weight neutral and would not exacerbate weight problems in this obese patient. The DPP-4 inhibitor linagliptin can be used at the full recommended dose regardless of the extent of renal impairment.

The addition of a GLP-1 RA is an option recommended by NICE when other recommended triple therapy combinations do not control blood glucose and is associated with weight loss, which can sometimes be considerable. However, this patient has moderate renal impairment and care should be taken to use a GLP-1 RA, which is indicated in this situation. If a GLP-1 RA is added, the dose of sulphonylurea should be reduced (with ulti-mately the aim of stopping this altogether) to reduce the risk of hypoglycaemia.

CASE STUDY 6.5: A 55-YEAR-OLD MAN WITH TYPE 2 DIABETES DIAGNOSED 6 YEARS AGO

- BMI 31 kg/m^2. Normal renal function and well-controlled cardiovascular risk factors, but recently diag-nosed with severe chronic obstructive sleep apnoea.
- HbA1c 8.0% (64 mmol/mol).
- Drugs: statin and anti-hypertensive agents, metformin 1000 mg bd.

Based on the observed phenotype, how does the guideline recommendation apply to this individual?

HbA1c is 8.0% on metformin monotherapy at close to maximal daily dose; therefore, treatment intensification is appropriate.

Are recommended therapies concordant with other conditions?

Agents that would promote further weight gain such as sulphonylureas, pioglitazone and insulin are not recommended as they could worsen the sleep apnoea.

According to NICE guidelines (NICE, 2015), GLP-1 RAs are not recommended dual therapy options, although a good case could be made here because of their ability to promote weight loss. DPP-4 inhibitors could be an option, but are weight neutral. An SGLT-2 inhibitor (or GLP-1 RA) is the physician's preferred option as it will not only improve glycaemic control but may also help with weight loss, which may be sufficient to improve the sleep apnoea.

EARLY AND INTENSIVE TREATMENT WITH INITIAL COMBINATION THERAPY

Type 2 diabetes is a silent disease for many years such that by the time of diagnosis a high proportion of β cells are already destroyed. This decline continues during the course of the disease resulting in progressive loss of glycaemic control often despite treatment with anti-diabetes agents. Until recently, most guidelines have proposed that additional glucose-lowering therapies are added to metformin in a stepwise manner when blood glucose control is inadequate. However, the stepwise treatment approach can result in serial failures to maintain normoglycaemia while the disease is progressing. In addition, intensification of treatment is often delayed resulting in long periods of hyperglycaemia and increased risk of vascular complications. It is clear that with the traditional stepwise approach to advancement of therapy, patients are not controlled in a timely fashion, and more than a third are not controlled at all (National Diabetes Audit, 2014–2015). Furthermore, even those who are controlled are subject to the progressive decline in β-cell function.

There is evidence that early and intensive blood glucose lowering by using initial drug combination therapy may preserve and improve residual β-cell function (Van Raalte et al., 2014). In addition, oral agents are now available (metformin and DPP-4 inhibitors) that in combination address many of the defects of type 2 diabetes with essentially no risk of weight gain or hypoglycaemia. Such a strategy may be particularly beneficial in the increasing number of younger individuals diagnosed with type 2 diabetes who will have a greater exposure to hyperglycaemia over a life time and therefore a greater risk of long-term complications. Such patients may also benefit from more stringent HbA1c goals, particularly because they are less likely to be suffering from comorbid conditions. There is a body of evidence, indicating that early, intensive treatment aimed at tight blood glucose control results in a legacy effect, so that benefits are maintained for many years, regardless of blood glucose levels later in the course of the disease (Ceriello, 2009; Holman et al., 2008).

The currently available oral anti-diabetes agents have different mechanisms of action. However, most (with the exception of SGLT-2 inhibitors and alpha-glucosidase inhibitors) exert their anti-hyperglycaemic effects through an insulin-mediated mechanism (e.g. increasing insulin secretion or improving insulin sensitivity, etc). As β-cell function declines with increasing duration of diabetes, these agents ultimately become ineffective, even in combination. To date, no anti-diabetes agent has been shown to arrest or reverse β-cell decline indefinitely in type 2 diabetes. Therefore, many/most patients with type 2 diabetes will ultimately need insulin to achieve their glycaemic targets. There are also data to suggest that intensive insulin treatment early after diagnosis may lead to long-term improvements in β-cell function. In a small, uncontrolled trial in 16 recently diagnosed patients, glucose was lowered to normal range by daily insulin injections within a time course of 2–3 weeks (Ryan et al., 2004). After the intervention, patients received diet therapy alone and seven remained euglycaemic at 1-year follow-up. The results of the Outcome Reduction With Initial Glargine Intervention (ORIGIN) trial indicated that insulin initiated early after a diagnosis of type 2 diabetes in combination with oral agents (not as a stepwise addition) resulted in a stable pattern of glycaemic control over the approximately 6 years of study (Gerstein et al., 2012).

Insulin treatment may be started at any degree of glycaemic control, even temporarily, according to the judgement of the treating physician, bearing in mind the risk to benefit ratio, for example, weight gain in overweight or obese patients and hypoglycaemia in frail elderly and or renally impaired patients. Many patients may initially be averse to early treatment with either oral combination therapies or insulin. However, they may be more accepting if the treatment is temporary and later results in less severe forms of disease that can be managed with lower doses of anti-diabetes agents. There are currently no studies that clearly address the comparative efficacy of initial combination therapy versus stepwise addition of therapy over time. Given that individuals with type 2 diabetes are heterogeneous in their clinical features and that it is a progressive disease, there is a clinical need for a personalised algorithm that covers these issues. At the very least, each individual step in these algorithms must be rapidly reviewed if HbA1c targets are not achieved.

ADVANTAGES OF A PERSONALISED APPROACH

There are a number of reasons for selecting a personalised approach to diabetes care. Guidelines for chronic conditions are generally based on clinical trials of highly selected participants, with many of the 'real-world' patients in general practice populations being excluded due to the presence of comorbidities or other factors. Strict HbA1c targets may not be achievable, or even appropriate, for many patients and should therefore be mutually agreed by the patient and physician. This recognises that not all patients have the same values or priorities. For example, patients who are older at diagnosis and who have coexisting conditions and a shorter life expectancy may warrant less stringent HbA1c targets. Revisiting the patient's preferences each time their clinical condition changes is also a routine part of diabetes treatment as the patient's priorities may change over time.

Patient non-adherence with treatment leads to adverse health outcomes and increased overall healthcare costs. When personalised therapies prove more effective and/or present fewer side effects, patients may be more likely to comply with their treatments. This also makes it less likely for clinical inertia to be an issue. These factors may have a major impact in chronic disease such as diabetes.

Finally, personalised care also has the potential to decrease healthcare costs by reducing inefficiencies such as trial-and-error dosing, hospitalisations due to adverse drug reactions, clinical inertia and reactive treatment.

REFERENCES

Ceriello A. Hypothesis: The "metabolic memory", the new challenge of diabetes. *Diabetes Res Clin Pract* 2009;86(Suppl 1): S2–S6.

Christian JG, Bessesen DH, Byers TE et al.; Clinic-based support to help overweight patients with type 2 diabetes increase physical activity and lose weight. *Arch Intern Med* 2008;68:141–146.

Dansinger ML, Gleason JA, Griffith JL, Selker HP, Schaefer EJ. Comparison of the Atkins, Ornish, Weight Watchers, and Zone diets for weight loss and heart disease risk reduction: A randomized trial. *JAMA* 2005;293:43–53.

Diabetes Prevention Program Research Group. Reduction in the incidence of type 2 diabetes with lifestyle intervention or metformin. *N Engl J Med* 2003;346:393–403.

Funck KL, Laugesen E, Høyem P, Fleischer J, Cichosz SL, Christiansen JS, Hansen TK, Poulsen PL. Low physical activity is associated with increased arterial stiffness in patients recently diagnosed with type 2 diabetes. *Am J Hypertens* 2016;29:882–888. pii: hpv197.

Gerstein HC, Bosch J, Dagenais GR et al.; ORIGIN Trial Investigators. Basal insulin and cardiovascular and other outcomes in dysglycemia. *N Engl J Med* 2012;367:319–328.

Holman RR, Paul SK, Bethel MA, Matthews DR, Neil HA. 10-year follow-up of intensive glucose control in type 2 diabetes. *N Engl J Med* 2008;359:1577–1589.

Inzucchi SE, Bergenstal RM, Buse JB, Diamant M, Ferrannini E, Nauck M, Peters AL, Tsapas A, Wender R, Matthews DR. Management of hyperglycemia in type 2 diabetes, 2015: A patient-centered approach: Update to a position statement of the American Diabetes Association and the European Association for the Study of Diabetes. *Diabetes Care* 2015;38:140–149.

Kanavos P, van den Aardweg S, Schurer W. *Diabetes expenditure, burden of disease and management in 5 EU countries.* London School of Economics; 2012. Available from: http://eprints.lse.ac.uk/54896/1/__libfile_REPOSITORY_Content_LSE%20Health%20and%20Social%20Care_Jan%202012_LSEDiabetesReport26Jan2012.pdf. Last accessed March 2016.

Lindström J, Ilanne-Parolla P, Peltonen M et al.; on behalf of the Finnish Diabetes Prevention Study Group. Sustained reduction in the incidence of type 2 diabetes by lifestyle interventions: Follow-up of the Finnish Diabetes Prevention Study. *Lancet* 2006;368:1673–1679.

National Diabetes Audit—2013–2014 and 2014–2015: Report 1, Care processes and treatment targets. Available from: http://www.hscic.gov.uk/catalogue/PUB19900/nati-diab-rep1-audi-2013-15.pdf. Last accessed February 2016.

National Institute for Health and Care Excellence. Type 2 diabetes in adults: Management. Clinical Guideline Update (NG28). Methods, evidence and recommendations; 2015. Available from: https://www.nice.org.uk/guidance/ng28. Last accessed March 2016.

Neeland IJ, Turer AT, Ayers CR et al.; Dysfunctional adiposity and the risk of prediabetes and type 2 diabetes in obese adults. *JAMA* 2012;308:1150–1159.

Ried-Larsen M, Christensen R, Hansen KB et al.; Head-to-head comparison of intensive lifestyle intervention (U-TURN) versus conventional multifactorial care in patients with type 2 diabetes: Protocol and rationale for an assessor-blinded, parallel group and randomised trial. *BMJ Open* 2015;5(12):e009764.

Ryan EA, Imes S, Wallace C. Short-term intensive insulin therapy in newly diagnosed type 2 diabetes. *Diabetes Care* 2004;27:1028–1032.

Tuomilehto J, Lindstrom J, Eriksson JG; for the Finnish Diabetes Prevention Study Group. Prevention of type 2 diabetes by changes in lifestyle among subjects with impaired glucose tolerance. *N Engl J Med* 2001;344:1343–1350.

Van Raalte DH, van Genugten RE, Eliasson B, Möller-Goede DL, Mari A, Tura A, Wilson C, Fleck P, Taskinen MR, Smith U, Diamant M. The effect of alogliptin and pioglitazone combination therapy on various aspects of β-cell function in patients with recent-onset type 2 diabetes. *Eur J Endocrinol* 2014;170:565–574.

Wei M, Gibbons LW, Kampert JB, Nichaman MZ, Blair SN. Low cardiorespiratory fitness and physical inactivity as predictors of mortality in men with type 2 diabetes. *Ann Intern Med* 2000;132:605–611.

7

Organisation of diabetes care

ROLE OF THE PRIMARY CARE TEAM IN MULTI-PROFESSIONAL CARE

An important consequence of a chronic condition such as type 2 diabetes is that it is not possible for any one healthcare professional to effectively provide the spectrum of care required. Integrating diabetes care with a team of professionals from a range of disciplines with different but complementary skills, knowledge and experience is critical to success and the prevention of both acute and chronic complications. Members of the team will vary according to the care required and because of other constraints such as resources, clinical setting and geographical location, but may include an ophthalmologist, podiatrist, dentist, dietician, diabetes educator and consultant diabetologist in addition to the general practitioner (GP) and local diabetes specialist nurse.

In the United Kingdom, approximately two-thirds of people with type 2 diabetes are managed entirely in primary care. The primary care team plays an integral role in integrating diabetes care and in ensuring that it is continuous and patient-centred at all stages of the disease. Many people with type 2 diabetes will also have at least one additional chronic health problem, and the primary care team also has the unique ability to provide continuity and coordination of care for patients with multiple chronic diseases.

As a patient's needs may change with time, the composition of the team may also need to change. Given the number of different healthcare professionals who will be involved in the care of a person with diabetes over their lifetime, maintaining a consistent approach to management can be difficult. The one constant is the person with diabetes, and they should be at the centre of the personalised management plan. The aim of integrating care is to refocus services around the individual with diabetes, removing barriers between specialties and organisations (integrated care = person-centred coordinated care). By working together, multi-professional teams can minimize patients' health risks by identifying problems early and initiating timely treatment so that the patient has the best possible outcome.

All team members have a role to play in providing consistent messages, which should reinforce the importance of metabolic control and effective management of other cardiovascular risk factors. This will include emphasising the value of a healthy lifestyle that includes physical activity and healthy eating. They can also emphasise the benefits of attending routine foot, eye and dental check-ups to prevent complications. The end result should be high patient satisfaction with care, good quality of life, improved health outcomes and ultimately lower healthcare costs.

Organizing high-quality care for the rapidly increasing number of people with type 2 diabetes is a major challenge worldwide. Although multi-professional care offers a more diverse range of skills and experience than a single healthcare professional can provide, the coordination of care can be challenging when delivered by multiple individuals in various settings, and it is important to ensure that there is neither unnecessary duplication nor gaps in service delivery and unacceptable delay. Coordination of care works best when there is a clearly identified person undertaking this role within the multi-professional team. In some cases, care coordinators may be directly involved in providing care, whereas in other cases, their role may be to facilitate care provided by other professionals.

The National Health Service (NHS) Five Year Forward View published in 2014, set out a new shared vision for the future of the

NHS based around new models of care. It emphasised that over the next 5 years (and beyond), the NHS would need to target the traditional boundaries between primary care and secondary care and community services, which often act as a barrier to the personalised and coordinated health services people require (NHS, 2014), and instead integrate care at all levels to optimise outcomes in people with type 2 diabetes.

Aims of integrated care

The aims of integrated care are as follows:

- To provide a high standard of specialised care for individuals with diabetes and their families from a multi-professional team
- To provide a greater range of seamless diabetes services closer to patients' homes
- To support those working in primary care to deliver first-class diabetes care
- To support and empower people with diabetes to manage their diabetes effectively
- To improve access to diabetes services
- To improve communication and closer working with GPs and other community services
- To provide education, training and support to the healthcare professional working in primary care

There are many ways of achieving integrated care, and the intensity of integration will vary according to individual circumstances and settings as illustrated in Figure 7.1 (Leutz, 1999).

For example, one solution may be the use of integrated community diabetes services to support primary care such as Intermediate Care Clinics for Diabetes (ICCD). Typically, these are community-based, multi-professional teams, working closely with general practices with the aim of delivering high-quality care nearer to patients. A number of these are already functioning across the United Kingdom. People referred are typically those with poorly controlled type 2 diabetes and/or cardiovascular risk

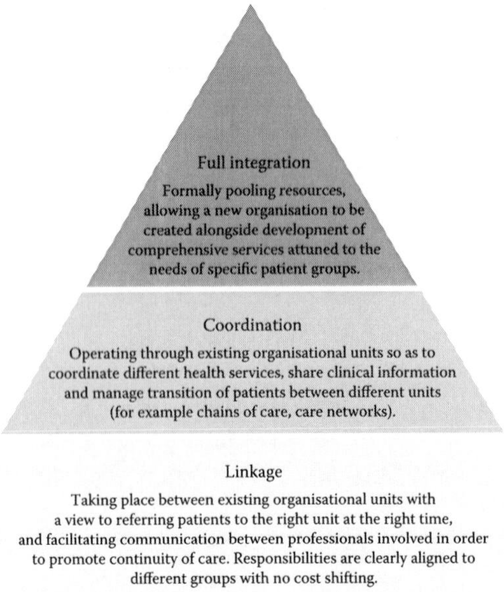

Full integration

Formally pooling resources, allowing a new organisation to be created alongside development of comprehensive services attuned to the needs of specific patient groups.

Coordination

Operating through existing organisational units so as to coordinate different health services, share clinical information and manage transition of patients between different units (for example chains of care, care networks).

Linkage

Taking place between existing organisational units with a view to referring patients to the right unit at the right time, and facilitating communication between professionals involved in order to promote continuity of care. Responsibilities are clearly aligned to different groups with no cost shifting.

Figure 7.1 Intensity of integration. (Leutz, W.N., *Milbank Quarterly*, 77, 77–110, 1999).

factors. Patients are managed by the ICCD team until the control of risk factors is achieved and then referred back to primary care. Such clinics have been shown to contribute to increased achievement of NICE targets for HbA1c, blood pressure and cholesterol in patients with diabetes, and both patients and primary care physicians have welcomed such enhanced service in the community (Wilson et al., 2014). Cost savings were not observed in a randomised, controlled trial of 49 general practices randomised to usual care or ICCD intervention in which patients were followed for 18 months (Wilson et al., 2014). However, cost savings may not be immediately obvious, as they often relate to the longterm burden of treating complications in secondary care and the effects on patients and their families of morbidity and premature mortality.

PERSONALISED CARE PLANNING

The aim of personalised care planning is to ensure that people with long-term conditions are given individual support to develop the knowledge, skills and confidence they need to effectively manage their health. It is a holistic approach that centres on listening to individuals, finding out what matters to them and what support they need, while taking into account their health, personal, family, social, economic, educational, mental health, ethnic and cultural backgrounds.

Care planning will vary depending on the complexity of a person's needs. For example, someone who has just been diagnosed with type 2 diabetes will have different needs to someone who understands and has accepted their condition, or someone who has diabetes-related complications.

As a minimum, a care planning discussion ought to focus on the following:

- Agreeing the individual's goals (e.g. I want to lose weight, stop smoking, get out more)
- Providing information (timely, relevant, ongoing)
- Supporting individuals to self-care, to take a more active role in their own health
- Agreeing on any treatments, medications or other services such as access to support groups or structured education programmes
- Agreeing any actions
- Agreeing a review date

Preparing for a care planning discussion

Good communication skills are crucial for optimising a care planning discussion and supporting individuals to self-care. The UK Department of Health has developed a range of materials to help healthcare professionals improve care for people with long-term conditions (NHS, 2011). The following questions are taken from one of healthcare professionals' information sheets and may prompt them to think about how they interact with individuals:

Do I communicate effectively?

Do I listen?

Do I support individuals to make informed choices?

Do I support individuals to access appropriate information?

Do I support individuals to develop skills in self-care?

Do I discuss risk?

Do I put aside my own health beliefs?

Do I view the individual in front of me as having expert knowledge in addition to mine?

Do I see the individual as a whole – not just concentrate on the individual's medical condition?

Am I supporting this individual to take control?

Do I ensure that those with complex needs are receiving coordinated care?

Do I strive to work across agencies and promote safe information sharing?

Do I ask individuals what they feel they need to better self-manage?

Do I ask individuals if they have any ideas as to the services they would like to be included in their plan?

When people recognize that they have an important role in self-managing their condition and have the skills and confidence to do so, they experience better health outcomes (Greene and Hibbard, 2012). With effective support and education, evidence shows that these skills can be developed and strengthened, even among those who are initially less confident, are less motivated or have low levels of health literacy (Hibbard and Greene, 2013). For the patient, being part of a multi-professional team that supports him or her and provides him or her with the right input at the right time can make all the difference between being in control of his or her condition or not.

In summary, it is vital that patients are central to all decision-making and care/management plans. This means agreeing with the individual what lifestyle changes are both appropriate and achievable. Agreeing realistic targets for glycaemic, blood pressure and lipid control are also important and will differ in different people. For example, an agreed HbA1c target for a younger, recently diagnosed, relatively uncomplicated patient of 6.5% (48 mmol/mol) should be both reasonable and attainable (ideally using drugs that do not cause weight gain or hypoglycaemia). The HbA1c target for an elderly person with long-standing type 2 diabetes who lives alone, has angina and has some renal impairment might be very different at, say, 7.5% (58 mmol/mol) or even 8% (64 mmol/mol). Similar considerations would need to apply for the other cardiovascular risk factors. The means to achieve these targets need also to be personalised as do measures of success.

The personalised/individualised approach to diabetes management, therefore, sees the patient and his/her needs as the prime focus for development of care plans. This is simply restating basic Hippocratic principles. Sometimes, these may be forgotten in the rush to embrace the rapidly developing science whilst forgetting the art of medicine!

REFERENCES

Greene J, Hibbard JH. Why does patient activation matter? An examination of the relationships between patient activation and health-related outcomes. *J Gen Intern Med* 2012;27:520–526.

Hibbard JH, Greene J. What the evidence shows about patient activation: Better health outcomes and care experiences; fewer data on costs. *Health Affairs (Millwood)* 2013;32:207–214.

Leutz WN. Five laws for integrating medical and social services: Lessons from the United States and the United Kingdom. *Milbank Quarterly* 1999;77:77–110.

NHS. Five year forward view 2014. Available from: https://www.england.nhs.uk/wp-content/uploads/2014/10/5yfv-web.pdf. Last accessed March 2016.

NHS. Improving care for people with long term conditions. Information sheet 1: Personalised care planning 2011. Available from: https://www.gov.uk/government/uploads/system/uploads/attachment_data/file/215946/dh_124048.pdf. Last accessed March 2016.

Wilson A, O'Hare JP, Hardy A, Raymond N, Szczepura A, Crossman R, Baines D, Khunti K, Kumar S, Saravanan P; on behalf of the ICCD Trial Group and the CCD Trial Group. Evaluation of the clinical and cost effectiveness of intermediate care clinics for diabetes (ICCD): A multicentre cluster randomised controlled trial. *PLoS One* 2014;9(4):e93964.

Index

Note: Page numbers followed by f and t refer to figures and tables, respectively.